THE EARLY IDENTIFICATION O
IMPAIRMENT IN CHILDREN

FORTHCOMING TITLES

Brain Injury Rehabilitation
A neuro-functional approach
Jo Clark-Wilson and Gordon Muir Giles

Writing for Health Professionals
Philip Burnard

Psychology and Counselling for Health Professionals
Edited by Rowan Bayne and Paula Nicholson

Occupational Therapy for Orthopaedic Conditions
Dina Penrose

Living with Continuing Perceptuo-Motor Difficulties
Dorothy E. Penso

Teaching Students in Clinical Settings
Jackie Stengelhofen

An Introduction to Communication Disorders
Diana Syder

Speech and Language Disorders in Children
Dilys A. Treharne

THERAPY IN PRACTICE SERIES
Edited by Jo Campling

This series of books is aimed at 'therapists' concerned with rehabilitation in a very broad sense. The intended audience particularly includes occupational therapists, physiotherapists and speech therapists, but many titles will also be of interest to nurses, psychologists, medical staff, social workers, teachers or volunteer workers. Some volumes are interdisciplinary, others are aimed at one particular profession. All titles will be comprehensive but concise, and practical but with due reference to relevant theory and evidence. They are not research monographs but focus on professional practice, and will be of value to both students and qualified personnel.

The Early Identification of Language Impairment in Children

Edited by
JAMES LAW
Lecturer in Child Language,
Department of Clinical Communication Studies,
City University, London

CHAPMAN & HALL
London · Glasgow · New York · Tokyo · Melbourne · Madr~

Published by Chapman & Hall, 2–6 Boundary Row, London SE1 8HN

Chapman & Hall, 2–6 Boundary Row, London SE1 8HN, UK

Blackie Academic & Professional, Wester Cleddens Road,
Bishopbriggs, Glasgow, G64 2NK, UK

Chapman & Hall, 29 West 35th Street, New York NY 10001, USA

Chapman & Hall Japan, Thomson Publishing Japan, Hirakawacho
Nemoto Building, 6F, 1–7–11 Hirakawa-cho, Chiyoda-ku, Tokyo 102,
Japan

Chapman & Hall Australia, Thomas Nelson Australia, 102 Dodds Street,
South Melbourne, Victoria 3205, Australia

Chapman & Hall India, R. Seshadri, 32 Second Main Road, CIT East,
Madras 600 035, India

Distributed in the USA and Canada by Singular Publishing Group
Inc., 4284 41st Street, San Diego, California 92105

First edition 1992

© 1992 Chapman & Hall

Phototypeset in 10/12pt Times by Intype, London
Printed in Great Britain by Page Bros, Norwich

ISBN 0 412 39340 9   1 56593 026 6 (USA)

RJ496
.L35
E29
1992

A catalogue record for this book is available from the British Library

Contents

Contributors

James Law, BA, MCSLT
Lecturer in Child Language,
Department of Clinical Communication Studies, City University,
London

Ros Herman, BA, MCSLT
Lecturer,
Department of Clinical Communication Studies, City University,
London

Rosemary Emanuel, MSC, MCSLT Dip (Aud)
Lecturer,
Department of Clinical Communication Studies, City University,
London

Carrie Pollard, RGN (HV)
The Lawson Practice, St Leonard's Hospital, London

Michael Crowley, CQSW
Lower Clapton Child Guidance Unit, London

Acknowledgements

I would like to acknowledge the clinical experience that I have gained from my work with language impaired children and their families. Although early identification can sometimes appear to be primarily a methodological issue, it is important that individuals do not get lost in the process.

I am very grateful to Drs Andrew Thomas, Martin Bax, and David Hall for their discussion of relevant matters (methodological and otherwise). I would like to thank Penny Roy for her reading of the manuscript and Mavis Taylor for her illustrations which will, I hope, serve to highlight one or two of the more salient issues.

Finally I would like to thank Jane for her thoughtful comments. She retained a level of objectivity about the text, something which I, at times, found difficult.

Foreword

What prompted James Law to devote a whole book to the identification of language impairment in children? Is there really enough to be said on the subject to fill 190 pages? No one who reads this book will be in any doubt about the answer. There is a wealth of information about the subject; the last twenty-five years have seen an explosion of research into that most fascinating of questions – how do children accomplish the extraordinary feat of acquiring their native language (or languages) in such a short time span, without special tuition, language laboratories or (in most cases) speech therapists?

Of course, the question is not new; it has fascinated thinkers for centuries. In 1705 the Moghul emperor Akbar Khan designed an interesting experiment, to investigate the nature of innate language. He incarcerated 12 babies in a castle, to be cared for solely by deaf and dumb nurses. When the children were 12 years old, they were brought before the Emperor's Court, to determine which language they had learned. Everyone was astonished to find that they did not speak any known language of the region, but communicated by gestures and signs. In 1992, although research on language acquisition is still in its infancy, perhaps we can at least claim that there have been some advances in methodology!

The ability to communicate clearly is highly prized in our Western culture. It is seen as the passport to success in business, the professions, and indeed in all walks of life. Not surprisingly, therefore, parents, health professionals and teachers are concerned about children who have difficulties in the acquisition of spoken language, fearing that they will find it difficult to compete in school and subsequently in the job market. Children of socially disadvantaged families are thought to be at particular risk. One result of this concern has been an increasing enthusiasm for earlier detection and treatment of speech and language problems. Many countries now incorporate some form of language screening into their routine child health programmes.

Perhaps the most important lesson to be learned so far in language acquisition research is that the process is very complex and that it is extremely difficult to tease out the various factors which might affect it. Not one challenge but a whole series confronts those who wish to detect and treat children with speech and language problems. They have to define the nature of the problem with sufficient precision to decide who does or does not have an impairment; develop a suitable means of detection; ensure that the detection programme reaches all children at risk; provide appropriate treatment facilities; and demonstrate to sceptical health or education planners that the whole exercise is cost-effective.

Pre-school language problems have largely been the province of health professionals, but we cannot continue to consider language impairment and early intervention only as health matters. They are closely linked to pre-school services of all kinds, including education and daycare. Language development is the responsibility of parents as well as professionals and more attention must surely be paid to the role of the family and to finding ways in which this role can be facilitated. Ultimately then, the debate on these issues will have to extend beyond the health professions; it involves fundamental questions of political emphasis and the structure of society.

James Law and his co-authors provide authoritative summaries of current knowledge and insight into this difficult field, although very wisely they do not attempt to provide any final answers. All health professionals with a responsibility for the community care of young children need to be familiar with the problems posed by language impairment and will find in this volume an accessible and well reasoned state-of-the-art account.

David Hall, FRCP
Consultant and Hon. Senior Lecturer in Child Health,
St George's Hospital and Medical school.

Introduction

James Law

Henry is three. His mother is worried that he is not like her other two children who are now four and six respectively. He is difficult to handle and uses only three recognizable words. The health visitor has focused on his sleeping difficulties. The general practitioner has told her that children 'grow out of it' and that she should stop worrying. The psychologist says he is within normal limits for his non-verbal skills. The speech therapist says he has a specific expressive language delay. On top of this his mother has been told that first children learn language more quickly, that if you don't speak to children enough they never learn language and that children who keep using their dummies have difficulty with their speech. Yet she has made every effort to speak to him and he stopped using a dummy around his first birthday. Henry had an ear infection when he was eighteen months old and she was told then that this could affect his reading later on. In short, Henry's mother is confused.

Speech and language problems are the most common of all preschool problems (Drillien and Drummond, 1983). Yet, as Henry's mother has found to her cost, there remains a great deal of uncertainty associated with the process of acquiring speech and language. Not surprisingly this uncertainty is often reflected in the understanding of parents themselves.

Kamhi (1988) picks out three examples of beliefs about early language development which are held by many parents and which will be familiar to most people who work with them. For example, parents will say that their children's first utterances are fully-formed words, Kamhi gives as his favourite examples 'flamingo' and 'succotash'. Clearly parents and linguists do not necessarily see eye to eye on what constitutes a word. Parents often maintain that the older sibling can understand a child whom others find unintelligible – the 'older sibling as interpretor myth'. Reviewing the evidence, Kamhi suggests that there is only very rarely a discrete shared language between children in a family. Finally, parents will often say that their child did not start speaking until five years and then went straight into speaking in sentences. Kamhi observes that, while the period between first words and complex structures may be very short, there is simply no recorded evidence that children bypass developmental phases. Where there is no pathology these beliefs are, as Kamhi observes, relatively benign. The problem arises once they are used as *post hoc* justifications for the fact that a child is experiencing real difficulties in learning to communicate.

The study of child language disorders has expanded considerably over the past fifteen years and it has become subsumed under a variety of different academic and clinical disciplines. Indeed the topic is considered the remit of those interested in neurology, audiology, aphasiology, paediatrics, psychiatry, phonetics, education, occupational therapy, physical therapy, psychology and, finally, speech pathology in the US and speech and language therapy in the UK. Some aspects of the subject clearly lend themselves to one discipline rather than another. Thus the transcription and analysis of language samples obviously falls within the remit of clinical linguistics. Others become the focus of interest for a range of different professions such that each angle sheds different light on the topic. Inevitably, the variety of interested disciplines has resulted in a multiplicity of interpretations of the causes and presentations.

As understanding of the conditions increases, so those involved look at ways of intervening to improve the situation of the children concerned. One step in this process is finding the best point in time to initiate clinical involvement. It is now relatively widely accepted that children who experience these conditions should be picked up as early in their development as possible. The difficulty is that many of the symptoms only manifest themselves clearly when the child is older and clinicians must ask whether it is not better to wait until the child is well into school before intervening (Stark and Tallal, 1981). From a census of all health districts in the UK, it is clear that those providing the service for preschool language impaired children consider that it is possible to identify language impaired children correctly before they are four (Law, 1991). Yet, to a great extent, this process remains an article of faith rather than one of proven value. Amongst others, Hall

(1989) has indicated that there is simply insufficient evidence to warrant the search for children with language problems, or indeed children with a great variety of other conditions. Given the resources necessary to carry out early identification programmes, this is an important point. Thus the issue of early identification, which grew out of assumptions and good intentions, is currently being subjected to increased scrutiny by those who have a responsibility for providing services.

This book has been written to draw together the principal issues related to early identification and screening of children with speech and language impairment. 'Early', in this context, is taken to be the preschool years. The book is intended for anyone working with the preschool child. This includes those with day-to-day responsibility for the care and education of children, notably nursery teachers and care staff; those who have responsibility for the identification of children with speech and language difficulties, especially paediatricians, clinical medical officers, health visitors, and practice nurses. It will also be of value to those working in the remedial field, particularly speech therapists, psychologists and teachers with specific responsibility for working with language impaired children. Finally, the book is intended for students of each of these disciplines.

It is important to note that the book is not primarily concerned with the identification of children that have secondary language impairments, that is to say those that have problems which are associated with another pervasive disorder such as autism or global developmental delay. Of course, the clear-cut categories common in the research literature are seldom immediately recognizable. Thus we speak of children with communication problems who have autistic features but for whom a placement in an autistic unit would not be appropriate. Similarly many language impaired children at three years present as being generally delayed. Yet we would hesitate at referring to them as such, until careful examination of their relative abilities had been made.

A frequent question which is raised regards the early identification of children from different language backgrounds. These children often prove especially challenging for those offering services to preschool children. Unfortunately there is usually too little known about language acquisition in the language groups of immigrant children to make generalizations as to the point at which difficulty reaches the level at which intervention is indicated. This book does not directly address this issue and the majority of references relate to anglophone services. Although there may be divergence in linguistic development between different languages, it is reasonable to assume that the same principals regarding early identification will apply. Those with a particular interest in this topic should find much of value in the text.

Finally, it would have been an impossible task to provide a definitive overview of services available to these children. The data available is too diverse to be easily interpreted. More important, perhaps, it is difficult to see what this would achieve in our attempts to unravel the complexities of the subject. Nevertheless, from time to time, reference is made in the text to specific examples of service provision. It is recognized throughout that looking for children with such problems is tackled in a great many ways in the UK and that the same is also true in the US, Canada, etc.

Chapter 1 gives a brief résumé of early communication development highlighting the role of the earliest interaction as the basis for subsequent development. The majority of children acquire the necessary skills with comparatively little difficulty. Indeed it has become something of a convention for those commenting on the subject to marvel at the achievement. Nevertheless there is variation in the population. Children seem to differ in the styles that they use to learn language. The literature relating to individual variation is discussed. In spite of this variation, a number of children do have particular difficulties in acquiring the necessary linguistic skills. Chapter 2 is devoted to describing the population which does not fall within the normal range. Much has been written which has taken the concepts of language delay/disorder, language deviancy, etc. for granted. Unfortunately this has often resulted in a confusing plethora of nomenclature which can baffle clinicians, students and parents alike. The chapter assesses the evidence that there are recognizable unfavourable patterns of communication development and looks at the evidence that children with speech and language problems simply get better anyway. If the difficulties do not persist there would be little reason for identifying these children in the first place.

One of the most confusing aspects of language impairment is that it is rarely a single entity. Parents who attend developmental clinics or speech therapy departments, doctors' surgeries or nurseries rarely complain that 'he is not speaking' without adding a list of other associated behaviours such as 'and he gets bored too quickly' or 'he never listens to what I say to him'. It is, as yet, unclear whether the language difficulty creates those other factors, whether in turn it is a function of them or whether they simply co-occur. Chapter 3 looks at the literature on the factors which have been shown to be connected to language impairment. These include other cognitive skills, play, behaviour problems, hearing loss and many others. It is important that all those who are in a position to identify these children are aware of these factors and are able to recognize the way in which they interact. Attempts at establishing aetiology have to date proved singularly unsuccessful. One alternative is the attempt to explain this interaction through the use of multivariate approaches. This is also discussed.

Two aspects of the child's development are considered in further detail. It is impossible to see children outside the context of their behaviour. It is now widely recognized that children who experience difficulties learning language frequently have difficulties relating to others and often come to be known as 'behaviour problems'. This frequently poses problems for clinicians being asked to distinguish between aspects of the child which are a function of behaviour and those which are a result of poor speech and language skills. Michael Crowley, a psychiatric social worker, examines the relationship between language development and behaviour in Chapter 4. He introduces two frameworks which are often used to look at children. The first is the psychoanalytic approach which provides insights into the motivation of the individual child. The second is the systems framework which aims to place the individual within the framework of the family. Language difficulties are discussed in terms of the effect they may have on family ecology.

One of the first aspects of the child in need of investigation from the speech therapist's or the paediatrician's perspective is the child's hearing. A great many children experience intermittent hearing loss in the first two or three years of their life and many of these go on to experience difficulties with their speech and language development thereafter. In fact, as Bishop and Mogford (1988) observe, the relationship between conductive hearing loss and language may be so intimate that treatment for the former may be dependent on difficulties with the latter. For this reason a specific chapter is included, related entirely to the identification and treatment of hearing loss. In Chapter 5 Rosemary Emanuel and Ros Herman, both speech and language therapists, give a clear and succinct description of the processes involved.

Chapter 6 turns to the basic principles underlying early identification. It adopts well-established medical criteria for screening and asks whether speech and language can ever be 'screened' in any formal sense. Other relevant concepts are also discussed.

Clinicians and teachers often ask whether there is any one test that accurately identifies the language impaired child. There are a great many different methods for identifying children with language impairment ranging from inspired clinical judgement, through to checklists, milestone charts and short tests. This variety often only serves to perpetuate the confusion. The chapter includes a review of a number of procedures. The role of the parent in early identification is also discussed.

In Chapter 7 Carrie Pollard, a health visitor, addresses the issue of early identification within the context of public health. Any programme of early identification will depend on the culture in which it is set. For this reason it is very hard to make generalizations which hold true for all countries. Indeed, for many countries, there is a conspicuous lack of literature. Of course this may mean that there is simply no service available. More likely it means that there is no consistent pattern to the system. Pollard looks at the international situation and discusses what can be learned from other countries. In particular she comments on the differences between the public system adhered to in the UK and the predominantly privatized system used throughout America. She goes on to discuss the importance of surveillance in the context of the changing structure of the nuclear family, a phenomenon common to all developed countries. Finally she offers an analysis of the different approaches to identifying language from the perspective of a consumer.

Although some authors (Lahey, 1990) have attempted to make a theoretical distinction between identification procedures and intervention, in practice the two are virtually inextricable. Indeed it has been suggested that screening should not be implemented unless there is both an accepted form of treatment and the resources available to carry it out. It is argued that it is unethical to highlight the need for referring a child without offering validated treatment. To do so would be to raise anxieties in the parent but do nothing to address them. At a more practical level, primary health care workers and teachers are unlikely to refer children for remediation if there is an inadequate service available for treating such children or if they feel that the treatment is unlikely to work. There is, as yet, no consensus as to appropriate treatment. Indeed much rests on the observational techniques used. As we shall see in Chapter 8, there is a need for considerable care in interpreting the results. There remains little evidence that one treatment works better for one clinical group than another. This, of course, refers back to the lack of coherence in describing the clinical groups themselves, introduced in Chapter 2.

The final chapter draws together the issues discussed in the text and sets them in a political context. While it is recognized that there is a specific 'scientific' method which may be applied to the evaluation of screening tests, it is clear that the issues relating to early identification are not confined to the efficacy of a single test. The book ends with a series of unresolved questions. It is hoped that the many health and education workers in the field will help contribute to answering these questions. It is only by addressing the correct questions in the first place and the professionals answering them together that Henry's mother, whom we met at the beginning of this chapter, will be able to make sense of the confused picture presented to her. In short this is an eclectic book about a topic which is of wide interest to a great many professionals working with the under-fives.

REFERENCES

Bishop, D. and Mogford, K. (1988) *Language Development in Exceptional Circumstances*, Churchill Livingstone, Edinburgh.

Drillien, C. and Drummond, M. (1983) *Developmental Screening and the Child with Special Needs*, Heinemann, London.

Hall, D. (1989) *Health for All Children*, Oxford University Press, Oxford.

Kamhi, A. (1988) Three popular myths about language development. *Child Language Teaching and Therapy*, **4**, 1–12.

Lahey, M. (1990) Who shall be called language disordered? Some reflections and one perspective. *Journal of Speech and Hearing Disorders*, **55**, 612–620.

Law, J. (1991) How are we screening our children? *Speech Therapy in Practice*, **7** (1), 16–17.

Stark, R. and Tallal, P. (1981) Selection of children with specific language deficits. *Journal of Speech and Hearing Disorders*, **46**, 114–122.

1

The development of early communication

James Law

This chapter identifies some of the principal issues arising out of the study of parent/infant interaction and the development of communication in children. Although the focus is on children who are not experiencing difficulties in learning to speak, the issues are pertinent to all aspects of early identification. One of the difficulties inherent in the study of early speech and language is the use of terminology. For this reason the chapter begins with an outline of some basic concepts. It then examines the sequence of communication development prior to speech and touches on the role played by hearing in the preverbal stage. Early linguistic development is then outlined and is followed by a discussion of the variation in the way children learn language.

TERMINOLOGY

Four interrelated components need to be identified. These may be itemized as follows.

1. Speech
2. Language
3. Communication
4. Intelligence

Each will be outlined in turn.

Speech

Speech constitutes verbal output. This includes both a physiological and a linguistic component. The former comprises **articulation ability** and includes structure of the oral space, and the resonators (larynx, etc.) together with the functional movement of the tongue, palate, etc. Articulation is conventionally transcribed phonetically. The latter comprises the sound or **phonological system** of the language used. Thus, all humans share the same articulatory mechanism, but different language groups make use of different sounds or phonemes. Every language has its own phonology and children acquiring that phonology may do so in slightly different ways according to the structure of the language concerned. Speech also includes the ability to coordinate volitional movements of the speech apparatus. This is termed **praxis** and is often associated with fluency of speech. It is important to recognize that praxis may include both articulatory and phonological components.

Language

Language is the symbolic system used to represent meaning within a culture. The relationship between the concept and the way in which it is expressed is essentially arbitrary. Conventionally six components of language are identified.

Phonology represents the sound system of a given language.

Prosody is the way in which meaning is conveyed through intonation and stress.

Syntax corresponds to the grammatical units used to convey meaning.

Morphology is the way in which words can change shape or be inflected within a given language – for example the addition of the '–ing' suffix for the present continuous tense in English.

Semantics represents the way in which meaning is stored and accessed. A distinction is sometimes made between referential meaning applied to the meaning implicit in the word itself and propositional meaning referring to the meaning derived from the combination of words.

Pragmatics are the rules governing the way in which language is used in a given culture.

Although these components are often isolated for the purpose of study, they are closely interrelated in the child. The nature of this relationship remains a matter for discussion but it is widely accepted that they may be represented in a model which includes both **input** – the capacity of the individual to decode the signal which is perceived – and **output** – the construction or encoding of a signal which will then be decoded by others. Decoding is synonymous with comprehension. **Verbal comprehension** is the term used for the process of decoding linguistic information.

Communication

Communication may be seen as an umbrella term which covers speech and language. Yet its application is not confined to speech and language. For example at a personal level it would include non-verbal behaviour and at a societal level would include all those factors which contribute to the transmission of culture. The study of communication is known as **semiotics** (see Halliday, 1978, for further discussion).

Bloom and Lahey (1978) have developed a model of language disorders in children which succinctly expresses the relationship between the component parts of communication (Figure 1.1).

In essence, these components interact in a meaningful way as the child develops. They become dissociated in certain circumstances resulting in restriction in the capacity to communicate (Chapter 2).

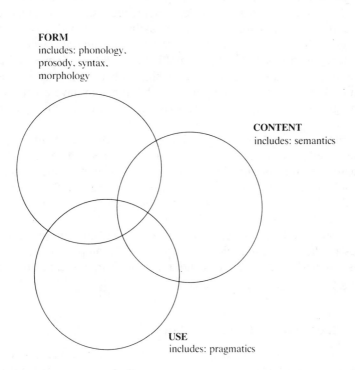

FORM
includes: phonology,
prosody, syntax,
morphology

CONTENT
includes: semantics

USE
includes: pragmatics

Figure 1.1 Bloom and Lahey's model of communication.

Intelligence

Intelligence has received extensive discussion throughout the literature (see Bee, 1989). The debate continues as to whether there is a single phenomenon 'intelligence' or 'g', as it is sometimes referred to, which may be measured in a unitary way, or whether there is simply a range of different skills which interact in an infinite number of ways. Certainly in clinical terms the latter view is more revealing and it may be that the discrepancy is more a function of the questions which researchers wish to answer than any real finite entity which will or will not be conclusively identified. In recent years, Gardner (1983) has put forward an appealing theory of 'multiple intelligences' which proposes a range of different intelligences – linguistic, musical, logico-mathematic, spatial, body kinesthetic etc., which operate within each individual. The saliency of each of these intelligences then depends upon the needs of the culture in which the individual develops.

In the study of language development, the issue of intelligence and the relative status of linguistic skills has been discussed at length (Yule and Rutter, 1987). While it is generally true that children with global developmental delays will have linguistic difficulties, the nature of the relationship between linguistic skills and other aspects of development in children who have no apparent global handicap of this type is far less clear. This will be discussed further in Chapter 2.

In the case of the young child, intelligence is conventionally measured in terms of developmental milestones and reactions to cognitive tasks of the type outlined by Piaget (see Piaget and Inhelder, 1969 and extensive discussion in Bee, 1989). Piaget outlined a number of basic stages to which reference is continually made. These are given in Table 1.1.

It can be difficult to separate out linguistic from cognitive abilities in the developing child. It would, for example, be hard to discuss a child's memory without referring to his capacity for language.

INTERACTION IN THE FIRST YEAR

It is sometimes assumed that speech and language are discrete entities which begin to emerge around the time of the first birthday. While it is true that they do appear at this time with astonishing predictability, it is impossible to examine that emergence without looking at the interaction of the child in the sensorimotor

Table 1.1 Cognitive stages identified by Piaget

Stage	Age	Description
Sensorimotor	Birth to 2 years	The baby relies primarily on sensory information and what may be done with objects which are experienced. Subdivided into six substages ranging from simple reflexes to the beginnings of thought.
Preoperational	2–6 years	By 18–24 months the child can represent objects to himself. He can classify objects and can take in others' perspectives. Fantasy play and primitive logic develop.
Concrete operational	6–12 years	The child's thinking remains tied to specific experience although there is now a capacity for powerful internal operations: addition, subtraction, class inclusion, etc.
Formal operational	12+ years	The child has an ability to manipulate the idea of events or objects in his head. He can imagine and think about things that he has never seen or that haven't happened. He can organize systematically and exhaustively and think deductively.

Adapted from Bee, 1989.

stage. Traditionally, researchers have emphasized the passivity of the child, Piaget's term 'sensorimotor' suggests a series of involuntary responses to the environment. The linguist Noam Chomsky has also emphasized this pacificity. He has illustrated the process of early language development as one in which the child develops language by simple exposure to a relevant linguistic environment in the way that a plant will grow given water. Yet, as the description of the very young child becomes increasingly sophisticated, it has become apparent that babies play a much more agentive role in the interaction process than has been recognized hitherto.

Some of the most elegant examples of work in this area have been produced by Trevarthen and his colleagues (see Trevarthen and Marwick, 1986; Trevarthen, 1989, for a review). There is evidence that the newborn has a preference for his mother's voice within a few hours of birth suggesting that the child may have developed this preference *in utero*. Within a matter of minutes of birth, babies can imitate pronounced facial expressions (tongue protrusions, etc.) and some may imitate simple hand movements. As Trevarthen notes, there are more subtle signs of readiness for human contact which have far-reaching implications. The newborn child has a capacity for communicating states of pleasure, curiosity, excitement, etc. and the parent learns to interpret these from the start, albeit with varying degrees of success. It is difficult to draw the boundaries between autonomous products of development and behaviours which follow from a learned response to the environment. Nevertheless it is possible to regard these very early communications in terms of their timing, form and energy. Trevarthen emphasizes the child's inbuilt motivation to communicate.

At around six weeks of age, the child's visual capacity improves dramatically and with it comes the capacity to focus on another's face. The information is then integrated with the auditory signal. This attention further elicits the marked pattern of vocalization in the parent which was originally termed 'motherese'. The fact that this pattern is thought to be the same in very diverse languages suggests that it is the child's contribution which plays a large part in determining the nature of this register. The result has been termed a **protoconversation** (Bateson, 1975) and it follows a very regular pattern. Each infant utterance lasts about two seconds, about the time that an adult takes to say a short sentence. Of particular interest is the fact that intervals between the beginnings of utterances suggest that parent and child seek to join with each other on the 'beat'. Trevarthen (1989) has observed that this beat speeds up from adagio (70/minute) to andante (90/minute) to moderato (115/minute) after a month or two of such protoconversations. Thus the parent and child learn to tune into one another and the child acquires the rudiments of 'use' and 'content'. The form is largely confined to coos or nuclear vowel sounds. Gradually the velar (/k g/) or glottal (/ŋ/) stop is integrated into the system closely followed by the introduction of lip and tongue sounds. Hand movements are often synchronized to these sounds and are often asymmetrical, being stronger on the right. This stage of mutual engagement has been termed **primary intersubjectivity** (Trevarthen, 1989).

After about three months, the child begins to explore the environment through active manipulation of objects. Developing muscle tone permits the child to track objects distant from the body, using sight and hearing. The features of the interaction noted above become stronger and the games that this elicits are consequently more active and more emotionally charged.

Trevarthen (1989) has identified universal parameters of the music used to entertain and soothe babies during this period. The quality (tension) and resonance of the mother's speech are regulated, as are the pitch and loudness, in harmony with the pulse of her breath control and articulation. The important point is that while the mother is entertaining the child she can only do so at a level which the child will accept. As the child reaches five months he begins to take more initiative as he becomes more self-aware. Trevarthen speaks of the baby 'becoming more expert at sharing jokes and showing off'. The play is full of 'metacommunications' – communications about shared, familiar subjects, facilitated by 'jokes' and the use of repeated silly faces. The child imitates more readily at this stage and the parent begins to teach appropriate tricks – clapping, etc.

The child then begins to develop learned fragments of behaviour or **protosigns** (Trevarthen, 1989), e.g. a funny expression in a given context. These are essentially arbitrary except that they have a shared meaning for the participants and a corresponding lack of response when presented to strangers. During this period the parent and child begin to share object play. Initially the child watches his mother, then begins to manipulate objects himself. Gradually they move towards a situation in which joint attention is held, and an object shared. After six months the child becomes aware that the games and learned activities are, to a certain extent, determined by the feelings of the other participant. He begins to check the response of the parent and uses 'emotional referencing'.

Trevarthen and Marwick (1986) have observed that the voice quality of the mother changes during this period. In the first few weeks there are relatively few feature changes in the voice which retains a predominantly breathy phonation. As the child develops so does the variation in the mother's voice. The child comes to recognize maternal intention from the vocal tone. This is essential because, as the relationship between parent and child develops, it is clear that the child does understand the parent's intention even though there is little likelihood that the intention is understood from the propositional content of what is said.

This leads, around nine months, to the infant beginning to develop a cooperative awareness. He learns that the object to which he has been attending has a meaning other than that dictated by his immediate experience of it. Once learned, this enables him to make reference of that object outside the context of the object itself. Simultaneously, the child begins to combine vocalization and gesture to signal wishes, feelings, purposes and experiences to his partners. This has been termed **protolanguage** (Halliday, 1975). It is not speech as such although some of the utterances become repeated family conventions and the child may crudely imitate the sound of certain words. It is at this stage that parents sometimes begin to impute overly sophisticated meaning into their child's utterances (see Introduction). This is the stage of **secondary intersubjectivity** identified by Trevarthen (1989).

From then on the child's communication skills develop dramatically with the onset of language development. Yet it is important to recognize that while it is possible to see this onset of language as being genetically triggered, its relevance rests squarely on the child's foregoing experience of primary and secondary intersubjectivity. Furthermore these early communication skills do not disappear with the onset of language. They may occupy a less salient position in terms of the detailed information that they are able to convey. Yet they continue to provide much of the structure for social interaction. A good example of this would be turn taking. It would be hard to imagine conversation without it and language is certainly an integral component of it. Yet the skills used here have their roots in these very early interactions.

THE DEVELOPMENT OF THE SELF

The development of intersubjectivity is inextricably linked with the growth of attachment in the first year. Stern (1985) speaks of the first year as a time when the sense of self develops. He describes four different senses of self. The **emergent self** forms between birth and two months, a sense of **core self** forms between two and six months. The **subjective self** forms between seven and fifteen months and a **verbal self** forms thereafter. The point is not that these 'selves' are stages through which the child must pass but, like the communication skills identified above, they operate in a cumulative fashion, the one adding to the others as the child develops. At the heart of his thesis is the assumption that infants are 'predesigned to be aware of self organising processes' and that given an appropriate environment they will progress in this fashion.

This appropriate environment is one in which the child learns to interact with others around him. This is especially true when, at around nine months, he becomes aware of the needs of others. This develops in part as a consequence of the child's developing self but also, in part, as a result of the role of the parent. Stern speaks of **affect attunement**, a process through which the parent goes beyond imitating the child to matching the child's output, whether behaviour or verbal output, in one of any number of modalities. Thus a child makes a sound which the mother echoes with a movement of her head and arm simultaneously. In other words the parent tunes into the feeling or intention of the child reflecting back to the child his or her own internal state. This allows the child to develop an awareness of the internal states of others, which in its own turn leads to the development of a 'theory of mind' which is such an integral part of the communication process.

THE DEVELOPMENT OF GESTURE

One skill which enables us to focus on the transition from non-verbal to verbal communication is that of gesture. The first intentional gestures of the second half of the first year have their roots in motor patterns developed from birth and are gradually interwoven with the emerging cognitive skills. By four to five months, the extension of the arm has been adapted to take in the child's perception of an object. By nine months, the child can systematically orientate and reach for a desired object. A great many other gestures – pointing, grasping, finger curling and spreading – emerge before they have any communicative intent and continue through until well after the onset of language. In fact, as Bates and colleagues have observed (1979), the movement patterns serve different functions at different periods in the child's development. One of these functions is communication. Once the motor patterns have been mastered, it is possible for the child to go on to use these sequences intentionally. Zanober and Martlew (1985) have identified four functional categories of communicative gesture – **expressive**, **instrumental**, **enactive** and **deictic**.

Expressive gestures are used to convey positive and negative emotional stress. Typical movements associated with positive emotions are the waving and flapping of arms, the clapping of hands, communicative smiles and face brightening, and excited stamping of feet. Negative emotions are signalled by sharp abrupt rhythmical movements of arms and legs, foot movements and movements involving the whole body. Often these movements are idiosyncratic initially but become replaced by more conventionally 'trained' gestures, such as clapping, around 18 months. Expressive gestures are often coordinated with vocalization from about ten months.

Instrumental gestures involve control of other people, either getting others to carry out particular tasks or rejecting advances. A typical example would be the infant raising his arms to be picked up but this category would also include the indicating of objects, or tapping on the mother's hand for attention. By ten months, children are using this type of gesture which rapidly become associated with a given word or sound. For many months, the child will continue to use both the word and the gesture as an indication of need.

Enactive gestures serve to build up shared meaning in given contexts and represent the actions and attributes of objects and people. These are often associated with given routines, e.g. washing, and become increasingly sophisticated as the child gets older. These activities are normally heavily modelled in the first instance but the child plays an increasingly prominent role. The gestures often directly mimic the activity itself – movements for unscrewing a jar or swinging on a swing. It seems likely that the use of such gestures is highly dependent upon the individual child, the emphasis placed on such movements within the family and indeed within the culture concerned.

Deictic gesture involves the child pointing at an object as a means of direct reference either at short range – proximal pointing – or some way away – distal pointing. This gesture first appears at about the nine month stage but is not fully operational until rather later. The largely referential nature of this type of gesture means that it is sometimes confused with the instrumental gesture identified above. Pointing plays an integral role in the development of joint attention throughout the second year of life. According to Zanober and Martlew (1985), pointing is accompanied by vocalization between 14 and 19 months, after which the vocalization takes over from pointing as the means of conveying deixis. Bates *et al.* (1979) have clearly associated this type of pointing with subsequent language abilities.

Of the four types of gesture, the first two – expressive and instrumental – emerge quite early and are internally driven, while the second two, enactive and deictic, require a more complex integration of skills and emerge more slowly. The latter pair allow for much greater communicative sophistication than the former. At this early stage, gesture provides one of the most effective methods of communication. In the majority of children the gesture then drops away to be replaced by speech. But it is important that speech is not necessary in order to be able to acquire language, as evidence from the deaf community shows all too clearly. By the time that the child has begun to integrate motor sequences and cognitive abilities into intentional gesture, the rudiments of language have already developed. And it is upon these building bricks that the more conventional external features of language, notably speech, are founded.

THE DEVELOPMENT OF HEARING

It is impossible to consider the development of early communication without also considering hearing. Our sense of hearing provides an important form of input before we are born. The auditory system is known to become responsive *in utero* from the 20th week of gestation. The developing child is thus able to hear sounds emanating from inside and outside the mother's body before birth, and can recognize and be soothed by the mother's voice soon after birth (see Northern and Downs, 1984, for an account of prenatal and neonatal hearing, and Appendix 1 for an outline of the ear and its function).

As the infant begins to explore his environment more actively, the information he receives from hearing is combined with information from other senses in learning about the world. For example, a soft toy dangling above the cot has certain visible characteristics which the child learns to recognize. When the infant reaches toward the toy and manages to touch it, the texture of the toy becomes more apparent. Touching the toy causes it to move and produce a tinkling sound. By integrating the look, feel, movement and sound of the toy, the infant begins to form a concept of the object. In the absence of normal hearing, the concept cannot be complete; the appropriate areas of the brain cannot be organized in response to sensations received by the ears; the infant's subsequent behaviour cannot be motivated by the fact that the toy produced a sound.

The newborn infant cannot 'close' his ears and so is constantly available to receive auditory stimulation. Early responses to sound such as arousal, pupillary dilation, crying or cessation of crying, and changes in cardiac activity (Eisenberg, 1976) have been used to investigate the development of auditory behaviour in neonates. Later responses are more readily observable. One such response, turning towards the sound source (which can easily be elicited at seven months of age), is utilized in an early form of hearing screening (see Chapter 5). The response is significant in helping the infant to identify the sound source, but it is important in later years in that it allows the child to locate potential dangers (e.g.

a car approaching from a bend). It also serves a useful function when participating in social groups and when listening conditions are less than ideal (e.g. in a noisy classroom). In these situations, locating and then facing the speaker allows the listener to focus his attention and also make use of visual information to understand what is being said.

Among the range of sounds to which the infant is exposed are some which he finds particularly fascinating, the sounds of speech. Indeed evidence from research suggests that neonates are predisposed to respond to linguistic aspects of speech (e.g. Eimas 1975). For example, even before learning the words of a particular language in his environment, the child is able to appreciate the expressive tone, or suprasegmental aspects, of speech used by the speaker (Spring and Dale, 1977). In the first few months of life, the infant can be seen to demonstrate this knowledge by responding pleasurably to a calm and pleasant sounding voice, but becoming distressed upon hearing an angry tone of voice. This early appreciation of intonation patterns and tone of voice forms the basis for the child developing responses to more complex patterns of social interaction; it is as important to interpret the way the message is expressed as it is to understand the words and the grammar used.

Evidence that children benefit from auditory exposure to language comes from studies of children who have been understimulated (see Chapter 3) and (more pertinent here) children who have or have had a hearing impairment. Children who have had the ability to hear language only in the first few months of life before becoming deaf have been shown to have significantly advanced language skills when compared with children who are deaf from birth (Greenstein *et al.*, 1976). Although the child has a natural capacity to learn language, he cannot develop this capacity to its full without being exposed to language from a very early age.

Hearing plays a dual role in the process of language acquisition; it enables the child to listen to language used by other people and to monitor his own sound production. The interaction between these two processes is evidenced in the range of sounds used in early babbling; as the child develops, the sounds he produces become restricted to those that he hears. Thus babbling from babies brought up in different linguistic communities becomes increasingly diverse, reflecting the sound systems of different languages to which the children are exposed.

The feedback which the child receives from hearing his own sound production is also rewarding and encourages the child to experiment with sound. The skills necessary for accurate sound production lag behind those for sound perception and discrimination. The auditory feedback loop enables the child to make the necessary fine adjustments to his own speech as increasing maturity allows the development of more precise articulatory control.

THE FIRST STAGES OF LANGUAGE

It is possible to describe comparatively discrete linguistic stages. For reference, an outline comparing linguistic and cognitive milestones is given in Appendix B. Barrett (1989) has identified three stages during the period of single word speech. The first of these is the period up to the time when the child has a productive vocabulary of ten words. Children vary as to when this stage has been achieved. Nelson (1973) found this to be between 13 and 19 months, with an average of 15 months. Usually these words are highly context bound and refer only to a given person or object in a certain situation. There is a corresponding tendency to under-extend the meaning of words. These first words, as already noted above, often lack real communicative intent. Rather they coexist with the child's activity, occurring alongside what the child is doing much like an independent action.

After this initial hesitation, words are usually acquired at great speed. The transition is marked by a move from 1–3 words per month to 25 words per month. This period is known as the **vocabulary burst** (Bates *et al.*, 1988). During this period, the infant continues to acquire context-dependent words while those that had previously been associated with a specific context become decontextualized and can be generalized to different situations. Alongside this trend comes the use of independent referential words which stand on their own, out of the immediate context, right from the beginning. This 'naming insight' (Barrett, 1989) is difficult to pin down in terms of age because such reports as there are suggest that there may be considerable individual differences.

As the child's vocabulary develops so does what he wants to use it for. Where the earliest intentions of the infant are relating to internal stages (e.g. reactions to objects) or directing the behaviour of others (e.g. requesting objects, directing attention), as the vocabulary increases so do the functions to which it is applied. The child learns to answer questions and to comment on what he hears around him. Similarly it enables him to take part in extended conversational exchanges.

By 19 months, children have usually acquired a vocabulary of fifty words (Nelson, 1973) and within two months of this most children have usually started combining words. These are of two forms; **pivot forms** with one word constant, e.g. 'allgone' or 'more', to which a new word is added and **categorical forms** in which words are in combination but not in any specified order. By 24 months, most children have acquired a considerable range of linguistic skills and are in the process of the **'grammar burst'**, a term used by Bates and her colleagues (1988) to refer to the phase when the child regularly combines words and starts to experiment with the form of language. Much of the rudiments of language, both in terms of expression and comprehension, are acquired by this stage. Between two and four, children acquire most of the adult forms of the language. In doing so they follow a fairly regular pattern of acquisition. Vocabulary during this period increases to several thousand words and the child is able to use language for a very wide range of purposes. The child continues to acquire syntactic rules although his or her system undergoes a number of readjustments as it aproximates to the adult model. In retrospect, the process may appear to the parents to be one of constant progress but, in reality, children acquire language in a series of spurts and plateaus, trying a range of new constructions at one moment and then spending long periods consolidating their gains.

Although the majority of grammatical rules are acquired by five years, children continue to develop different constructions – e.g. the passive or rules related to the asking of indirect questions – well into the school years. Furthermore their 'use' of language develops with their capacity to engage in sophisticated discourse with others around them. Most authors are now reluctant to tie specific grammatical constructions to specific ages because it has been shown that the age, although not usually the order of acquisition, is subject to considerable variation. This is central to the whole topic of early identification and for this reason the next section addresses the issue of variation in language acquisition.

VARIATION IN CHILD LANGUAGE ACQUISITION

Anyone working with young children knows that language performance depends on the circumstances in which the language was elicited. Wells (1986) found that children's language varied according to the different contexts in which they were interacting. For example, in play the child's verbal output depended on whether the adult was present or not. When the adult is absent, children use more statements to one another but fewer requests and responses. When joining in, the adult invariably employed more question forms, resulting in a shift on the child's part to response forms. Yet if this was the only type of variation which children presented, the task would be confined to obtaining an optimum language sample.

Bates et al. (1988) have noted a number of areas of variation in the rate at which children learn language. For example they point out that evidence from different languages indicates that there are differences in the way that both phonology and syntax are acquired. This may occur at the one-word stage, for example Turkish children sometimes begin to produce verb and noun inflections before they start putting words together. But the differences are most marked after 20 months of age, when grammatical development has already progressed considerably. The same authors also note differences in rate of development in phonology, in comprehension, single word production and in word combinations and in a number of the features of early grammar. To take an example, single word production varied from 0–52 words at 12 months (mean = 11.9), while at 28 months the variation was from 20 to 674 words (mean = 379.8) (Bates et al., in press).

Wells (1986) carried out a large study of the expressive skills of a representative study of children in Bristol, UK. He went to great lengths to obtain valid language samples from the children concerned, fitting each child with a radio microphone. He identified further variation between the subsystems of language, notably syntax, semantics and pragmatics. The correlations decreased between 42 and 60 months, suggesting that variation between the basic components of language increases with age. Wells concludes from this evidence that the older the child, the less suitable the use of single-skill measurements is likely to be.

In 1973 Nelson published a monograph following eighteen children longitudinally from approximately one to two years of age – i.e. through the one-word stage. She identified two discrete styles within this comparatively small group. The first used what she termed a **referential style** (i.e. with vocabularies with a high proportion of common object names) and an **expressive style** (heterogeneous vocabularies containing a wide variety of different classes of words, and including social expressions). After twenty years of further investigation these two styles have proved remarkably robust. For example Bates and colleagues (Bates et al., 1988; Bates et al., in press) repeat this basic dichotomy although the

15

terms used have changed. They identify two groups of children, the first **analytic**, the second **holistic**. The 'analytic' approach involves the child breaking language down into small units, and working out the relationships between these units before attempting a synthesis. This pattern manifests itself from babbling in which they tend to use short and consistent consonant–vowel segments, to first words where the child concentrates on object naming, to first word combinations which often appears as rather telegrammatic with function words and inflections eliminated. By contrast the 'holistic' child seems to adopt the opposite strategy, using relatively large global chunks which are only later broken down into units. Again, this approach seems to run through all levels of language development for the child in question. Of course, both styles are necessary for language development to take place but children may differ in the degree to which they adopt one style or another.

Reasons for such stylistic differences are, as yet, unclear. Wells (1986) suggests that there may be inherited family differences in the way that children learn language, although he is very cautious as to the nature of that relationship. Similarly the issue of the relationship between personality and the pattern of language development is one which has been raised but as yet relatively little is known about it. A temperamentally passive child may be less responsive than an active child and this may determine the nature of the linguistic stimulation which is received. It is logical that there should be continuities between the behaviours described by Trevarthen (1989) and Stern (1985) and subsequent linguistic performance but the link needs further investigation. The role of intelligence, to which reference has already been made, is likely to affect language learning strategies. Indeed Bates *et al.* (1988) discuss the possibility that the analytic child may be simply of higher intelligence, whereas the holistic child knows that repetition serves the communication function of cohesion, but takes longer to effectively analyse the individual units. There are clear parallels here with the 'echolalic' behaviour of the delayed child. However Bates *et al.* (1988) point out that this association is far from clear, suggesting rather that the different styles perform different functions. It may be the linguistic input which determines the relative emphases.

The effects of the gender of the child in relation to style differences have received considerable discussion in the literature. Initially girls were thought to develop language more quickly than boys but this evidence has been qualified in recent years and it has been suggested that it was child-rearing practices rather than the gender itself which was important. By contrast recent evidence has suggested that associations are either non-existent (Bates *et al.*, 1988) or slight (Wells, 1986). Furthermore, where they do occur they relate more strongly to the way in which the adult speaks to the child, not the other way around. Thus greater proportions of sequences of conversation were identified in the play sequences of boys but in helping or general activity activities of girls.

Another possible explanation is that variation is a function of specific mechanisms. Three such mechanisms have been identified by Bates and her colleagues (in press).

1. An analytic mechanism which segments the input, extracting invariant features and establishing patterns of correlation between sound and meaning. When present this mechanism yields high comprehension and is strongly associated with other aspects of non-verbal cognition.
2. A fine motor control mechanism that is partly responsible for turning patterns of analysed and comprehended speech into expressive language. This mechanism is closely associated with gestural ability and is not specific to language.
3. A memory device that permits storage and retrieval of large input patterns (which may or may not be specific to the speech channel); individual differences in 'language style' reflect the degree to which this mechanism develops ahead of or behind the analytic and motor devices (1 and 2).

There is, therefore, some considerable evidence for the variation both in terms of rate and style of language development. Great care has to be taken in making general statements about language development in terms of milestones, etc. This makes the task of those interested in the early identification of children with language impairment particularly difficult. If too little is known about variation in the population then judgement as to pathology on the basis of standard scores on individual tests is very difficult. Yet it is worth bearing in mind Well's comments on the subject

'At the present time, however, the weight of the evidence suggests that differences between children are best thought of in terms of minor deviations that branch off from and rejoin the main thoroughfare rather than as separate independent routes'

Wells 1985, p. 335.

SUMMARY AND CONCLUSIONS

The following points may be extracted from the foregoing discussion.

- The preverbal infant is motivated to be a good communicator, so that by the time language comes 'on line' at around the first birthday, most of the basic capacity to use it has already been developed. This requires a complex synthesis of cognitive processing, sensory information and affective development.

- Although it remains unclear as to how 'intentional' the infant is in his early interactions, it is clear that the parent is only able to determine the quality of the interaction on the child's terms. The issue of the extent to which the parent can actively interfere with the child's language acquisition at this stage remains unclear.

- Although the course of language development has now largely been mapped out, there is evidence of variation in both the rate and the style with which the necessary skills are acquired. There is, as yet, no comparable evidence for rate and style differences in communication in the first year of life. It remains unclear what impact these differences may have on subsequent performance.

Any attempt to identify children who have marked language difficulties must take communication into consideration alongside language. Furthermore it must provide a systematic way of differentiating between variations of the type outlined above and variations which are likely to cause significant problems. As we shall see in Chapter 2, closer examination of a number of different populations shows that a proportion of children do find the process of language acquisition especially difficult although the delineation of this group proves immensely problematical. Given the complexity of the interaction between the different components identified in the discussion above, this is hardly surprising.

REFERENCES

Barrett, M. (1989) Early language development, in *Infant Development*, (eds A. Slater and G. Bremner), Lawrence Erlbaum, London, pp. 211–41.
Bates, E., Benigni, L., Bretherton, I. *et al.* (1979) *From Gesture to the First Word*, Academic Press, New York.
Bates, E., Bretherton, I. and Snyder, L. (1988) *From First Words to Grammar*, Cambridge University Press, Cambridge.

Bates, E., Thal, D. and Janowsky, J. S. (in press) Early language development and its neural correlates, in *Handbook of Neuropsychology, Vol. 6, Child Neurology*, (eds I. Rapin and S. Segalowitz), Elsevier, Amsterdam.

Bateson, M. C. (1975) The Epigenesis of Conversational Interaction: a personal account of research development, in *Before Speech* (ed. M. Bulowa), Cambridge University Press, Cambridge, pp. 63–78.

Bee, H. (1989) *The Developing Child*, Harper and Row, New York.

Bloom, L. and Lahey, M. (1978) *Language Development and Language Disorders*, Wiley, New York.

Eimas, P. D. (1975) Speech perception in infancy, in *Infant Perception: From Sensation to Cognition Vol. 2*, (eds L. B. Cohen and P. Salpatek), Academic Press, New York, pp. 193–231.

Eisenberg, R. B. (1976) *Auditory Competence in Early Life*, University Park Press, Baltimore.

Gardner, H. (1983) *Frames of Mind: The Theory of Multiple Intelligences*, Basic Books, New York.

Greenstein, J. M., Greenstein, B. B., McConville, K. *et al.* (1976) *Mother Infant Communication and Language Acquisition in Deaf Infants*, Lexington School for the Deaf, New York.

Halliday, M. (1975) *Learning How to Mean*, Edward Arnold, London.

Halliday, M. (1978) *Language as Social Semiotic*, Edward Arnold, London.

Nelson, K. (1973) Structure and strategy in learning to talk. *Monographs of the Society for the Research in Child Development*, **38**, (1–2 Serial no. 149).

Northern, J. L. and Downs, M. P. (1984) *Hearing in Children*, Williams and Wilkins, London.

Piaget, J. and Inhelder, B. (1969) *The Psychology of the Child*, Basic Books, New York.

Spring, D. R. and Dale, P. A. (1977) Discrimination of linguistic stress in early infancy. *Journal of Speech and Hearing Research*, **20**, 224–232.

Stern, D. (1985) *The Interpersonal World of the Infant*, Basic Books, New York.

Trevarthen, C. and Marwick, H. (1986) Signs of motivation for speech in infants, and the nature of a mother's support for the development of language, in *Precursors of Early Speech*, (eds B. Lindblom and R. Zetterstrom), Macmillan, Basingstoke, Hants, pp. 279–308.

Trevarthen, C. (1989) Signs before speech, in *The Semiotic Web*, (eds T. A. Sebeok and J. Umiker-Sebeok), Mouton de Gruyter, Berlin, pp. 689–755.

Wells, G. (1986) Variation in child language, in *Language Acquisition*, (eds P. Fletcher and M. Garman), Cambridge University Press, Cambridge, pp. 109–39.

Yule, W. and Rutter, M. (1987) *Language Development and Disorders*, MacKeith Press, Oxford.

Zanober, B. and Martlew, M. (1985) The development of communicative gestures, in *Children's Single Word Speech*, (ed. M. Barrett), Wiley, London, pp. 183–215.

2

What is language impairment?

James Law

In the preceding chapter we examined the prelinguistic processes thought to be common to all children, noting both the consistency which children seem to show in the acquisition of communication skills and the range of potential variation in the style of that acquisition. This chapter examines the classification of children who have difficulty in mastering these building blocks of language and who consequently fall outside what may be considered the 'normal' range. We noted at the beginning of the Introduction that language problems are generally considered to be one of the most commonly occurring difficulties in preschool children. This chapter begins by looking at just how common these difficulties are. It goes on to look at the way these difficulties have been classified, paying particular attention both to the concept of specific language impairment and to the distinction between language delay and language disorder. It is impossible to look at the subject without referring to the natural history of language difficulties. So the extent to which these problems persist is examined at the end of the chapter.

PREVALENCE

Prevalence refers to the total number of cases in a given population at a given time. By contrast, **incidence** refers to the number of new cases of a condition occurring in a given period. The two are obviously related but prevalence is not simply a question of summing the number of new cases and adding them to an existing total. The number of those children whose communication difficulties have resolved spontaneously or for whom intervention has proved effective need to be excluded.

A great many studies have been carried out purporting to examine the prevalence of speech and language problems. In many cases the divergence in the figures given is quite baffling. There are two principal reasons for this. On the one hand, there is a lack of consensus as to the degree of severity warranting clinical attention. Terms such as mild, moderate and severe are used without adequate definition. On the other hand, the imprecise categorization of different types of language impairment makes direct comparison between studies difficult. The results, such as they are, indicate three levels of difficulty although it should be recognized that this classification is also subjective. Examples of studies within each category will be given and the variability between them will be discussed.

The most severe cases

Ingram (1963) found 0.071% and 0.075% with 'severe language retardation' in Edinburgh and Aberdeen respectively. Rutter, Tizard and Whitmore (1970) similarly found 0.08% of children with 'specific developmental disorder of language'. These figures suggest a level of consensus for the more severe disorders.

Pronounced cases

Five studies have specifically targeted three-year-olds. Randall *et al.* (1974) found nine out of a sample of 160 (5.6%) to be 'severely language retarded'. This they defined as having a standard score below −2 standard deviations on a scale of expression, comprehension or articulation. Fundudis, Kolvin, and Garside (1979) studied a screened population of 3300 three-year-old children in Newcastle, England, and identified 4% with moderately or severely retarded speech. In Dunedin, New Zealand, Silva, McGee and Williams (1983) looked at 1027 three-year-olds and found a total of 7.6% with delays in expression and comprehension. Richman, Stevenson and Graham (1982) examined a screened population of 705 children in the London Borough of Waltham Forest and found 3.1% with 'general expressive language delay'. Finally, Bax, Hart and Jenkins (1983), looking for language impairment in children at two years, three years and 4½ years, found that the proportions changed across time. Their results are presented in Table 2.1.

Table 2.1 Children presenting with poor language development

Age	No.	% with problems	Definition of problem
2 years	296	17%	Possibly abnormal
		5%	Definitely abnormal
3 years	323	12%	Possibly abnormal
		8%	Definitely abnormal
4½ years	269	7%	Possibly abnormal
		5%	Definitely abnormal

From Bax, Hart and Jenkins, 1983.

Less pronounced but nonetheless identifiable difficulties

A study in the Ottawa–Carleton region in Canada (Beitchman *et al.*, 1986) examined a population of 1655 five-year-olds to establish what proportion had speech impairment, language impairment or both together. Furthermore they used standardized measures and compared the numbers when cut-off scores of −1 and −2 standard deviations were used. The results are given in Table 2.2.

Table 2.2 Numbers of five-year-olds with speech and language impairment

Category	% at −1 standard deviations	% at −2 standard deviations
Speech	6.4	6.1
Language	8.04	1.8
Speech and language	4.56	1.7
Total	19.00	9.6

From Beitchman *et al.*, 1986.

Interpretation of the prevalence figures

- The numbers are highly dependent on the criterion used. Thus the more severe the condition sought and the more specific the skill under examination, the smaller the number identified. By contrast, definitions which include speech and those which attempt to identify children with milder problems inevitably identify more children.
- The numbers are also dependent upon the age at which the skills are assessed. In terms of the milder cases, at least, the numbers tend to decrease with age.
- Variation may be a function of the original screening test adopted. For example, the differences between the four

studies of three-year-olds may have been a function of the methods used for identifying the children. The Fundudis study (1979) asked health visitors to identify children who were not stringing three words together into a sentence to make some sort of sense. In Dunedin (Silva *et al.*, 1983) there was no screening measure as such because each child was assessed using the Reynell Developmental Language Scales and a cut-off of the fifth centile was adopted. In Waltham Forest (Richman *et al.*, 1982) part of the expressive section of the same test was used. In the Bax study (1983) the authors used a clinical judgement which had previously been validated against the Reynell Developmental Language Scales (Reynell and Huntley, 1985), such that children definitely failing scored below -1.5 standard deviations (Bax *et al.*, 1980).

- Variation in these figures may reflect real differences in the populations concerned, Silva *et al.* (1983), for example, admit that their sample was slightly skewed in favour of more privileged groups, while it would be fair to say that the Bax *et al.* (1983) group was probably skewed the other way. The authors of the Waltham Forest study (Richman, Stevenson and Graham, 1982) maintain that they chose the district in question precisely because in demographic terms it was representative of the country as a whole.

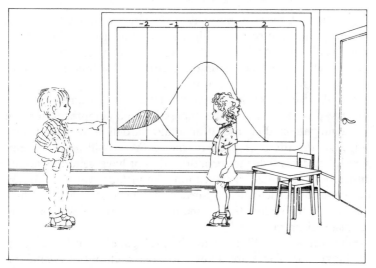

Where abouts do you come?

- The use of standardized tests in itself poses problems. The nature of the standardization procedure means that 2.8% of any population will score below −2.0 standard deviations below the mean; the equivalent figures for −1.5 standard deviations and −1 standard deviations are 6.68% and 15.87% respectively. To use tests which have been standardized necessarily suggests a circularity. In other words, you are likely to find the proportion you are looking for. It should be noted that not all the figures above did come from standardized assessments. Barker and Rose (1984) have noted that in many medical conditions, the normal distribution is naturally skewed so that there is an abnormally high number of clinical cases.

THE DESCRIPTION AND CLASSIFICATION OF LANGUAGE IMPAIRMENT

The *Diagnostic and Statistical Manual of Mental Disorders* (1980) provides a definitive classification system widely used in the United States. It includes under Axis II 'Specific Developmental Disorders', **315.31 Developmental Language Disorder**, which in turn is divided into three groups

1. Failure to acquire any language
2. Acquired language disability
3. Developmental language disorder

The first of these is normally associated with severe mental handicap, and the second with trauma or neurological disorder. Both could be considered language disorders secondary to a clearly defined medical condition. Neither fall within the remit of this book as outlined in the Introduction.

The third category is further subdivided into **expressive type**, and **receptive type**. Although expression and comprehension are frequently affected in cases of mental retardation, developmental language disorder, as used in the DSM classification system, clearly indicates that these children do not have general learning difficulties. The DSM classification also includes category **315.39 Development Articulation Disorder** in which speech difficulties cannot be attributed either to mental handicap or developmental language disorder.

However we are still left with the problem of what it is that we are looking at. There are, in essence, two methods of identifying the difficulty. These are as follows.

1. Defining the population in terms of the 'normal' population. This relies on the use of standardized testing procedures. This allows us to make accurate comparisons with other children. The problem is that the tests themselves do not determine what level constitutes a problem. Snyder-McClean and McClean (1987) and Lahey (1988) estimate a figure of 6.5% with difficulties. This corresponds to a level of −1.5 standard deviations referred to earlier. Clinically this seems to be a reasonable solution to the problem of where to apply a cut-off point. Yet what does this mean in terms of specific linguistic behaviours? Once an agreed level of acceptability is reached, it should technically be possible to reintroduce this into data samples which have examined the different ages at which populations of children acquire certain forms. By way of illustration, the data for the acquisition of linguistic functions taken from the Bristol Study (Wells, 1985) are adapted and presented in Appendix C. Similarly, the age at which it would be possible to predict that 90% of the population would have acquired certain phonological processes and speech sounds, are included in Appendix D. But before this approach can be usefully adopted it needs to be shown that, without intervention, this group is more likely to have persistent difficulties than a group with less pronounced difficulties. Although intuitively this would seem to be correct, it has yet to be shown to be the case.

2. Defining the population in terms of clinical symptomatology. Clinical evidence suggests that a given group of children have a poor prognosis and that therefore this group should be identified. This is comparatively easy if we describe the performance of children who have speech or language difficulties associated with other more clearly defined medical conditions − severe mental handicap or cleft palate, for example. The problem comes when speaking of children in the normal population who have no clinical features with which to identify them, other than their communication. In such circumstances we have to make clinical judgements in the context of the range of variation identified in the previous chapter. The difficulty here is that for symptomatology to be seen as such it must be possible to show that the classification can be reliably made.

In the final analysis, these two approaches should identify the same children. Despite the variation noted above, there is some indication that this may be the case. It is interesting, for example, that the 19% figure identified by Beitchman *et al.* (1986) corresponds to the figure given by Morley (1957) from a study carried out thirty years earlier, in Newcastle, UK, with much less clearly defined parameters. The subject is further confused by the plethora of terms used to describe different types and presentations of language impairment. There have, for example, been a number of attempts to introduce neurological terminology, e.g. congenital aphasia and developmental dysphasia. Although there is now some indication of abnormal cerebral activity in some cases, such terms are not generally considered appropriate for more than a narrow band of children presenting with very low levels of language.

Ingram (1972) looked forward to the day when 'classification will primarily be on the basis of linguistic and phonetic criteria' and there is no doubt at all that advances in linguistics in the 1970s highlighted the importance of a variety of features of child language. There are now extensive systems available for describing language in terms of linguistic features (Crystal, 1981). Some authors have attempted to define a range of subcategories on the basis of an interaction between psychological and linguistic characteristics. Aram and Nation (1975) used factor analysis to examine a group of 47 children (aged 3 years 2 months to 6 years 11 months) with developmental language disorders and identified six patterns of language performance based on high and low performance on three factors. The factors identified were

1. Comprehension
2. Formulation
3. Repetition

The patterns identified in the context of these factors were as follows.

1. **Repetition strength**: These were children with a high capacity for syntactic and phonological repetition but a lower comprehension ability.
2. **Nonspecific formulation–repetition deficit**: These children presented with poor repetition and syntactic formulation with relatively sound comprehension. Their performance on all language tasks was low.
3. **Generalized low performance**: This pattern represents a uniformly low performance on all tasks.

4. **Phonological comprehension–repetition deficit**: These children had difficulties which were largely confined to their phonological abilities.
5. **Comprehension deficit**: These children performed at a high level on repetition and formulation tasks but at a comparably lower level for comprehension.
6. **Formulation–repetition deficit**: These children performed at a higher level for comprehension and a correspondingly lower level for both formulation and repetition tasks.

The authors found that the younger the child the more generalized the effect of the language disorder. Thus group three were the youngest while group four were the oldest. This is in line with the finding from Wells (1986), identified in the previous chapter.

More recently, an attempt has been made to fuse linguistic and neurological classification systems (Rapin and Allen, 1987). These authors offer a classification system for preschool children with specific language difficulties.

Verbal auditory agnosia or word deafness, characterized by the almost complete inability to comprehend language through the auditory channel.

Verbal dyspraxia, characterized by effortful speech and poor phonological development. Comprehension is within normal limits.

Phonological programming deficit syndrome, characterized by low intelligibility although the amount that is said corresponds to expectations for the age of the child. A much less pronounced disability than dyspraxia. Comprehension is not affected.

Phonological syntactic deficit syndrome, characterized by low intelligibility and a correspondingly reduced syntactic output. Comprehension may also be affected.

Lexical syntactic deficit syndrome, characterized by normal phonological development, but poor word retrieval and poor use of connected speech. These children have particular difficulties reconstructing story sequencies.

Semantic pragmatic syndrome, characterized by slow acquisition of language and when it does come, it presents in a highly bizarre fashion. Although these children may perform adequately on structured comprehension tests, they often make arbitrary associations in conversations.

A similar classification system has been identified by Bishop and Rosenbloom (1987) but it still remains to be seen whether necessary and sufficient conditions can be generated to place children unequivocally in one group or another. The pattern which emerges is one of such diversity of difficulties, on the one hand, that it is difficult to see how any two children can be satisfactorily compared. Yet, on the other hand, authors such as Beitchman (1985) and Bishop and Edmundson (1987b) are increasingly stressing an underlying neurodevelopmental delay of which language is the more prominent if not the only manifestation. Given the evidence for associated difficulties, which we will consider in Chapter 3, this is an appealing theory.

SPECIFIC LANGUAGE IMPAIRMENT

In the classification outlined from the D.S.M. III, language disorders came under the category of 'specific' problems. This effectively means that it applies to language rather than other aspects of the child's abilities. 'Specific language impairment' or s.l.i. is conventionally defined by exclusion. Thus, children with s.l.i. are distinct from those with a more general language impairment because they are said to be of normal intelligence, to have no frank neurological symptoms, to have no hearing loss, to have no primary emotional disorder and not to have a predominant environmental disadvantage. Clearly, there are children whose language skills are markedly below their cognitive skills but for whom there is no obvious explanation for their difficulties. Yet it has proved difficult to provide the necessary and sufficient conditions for children to be included in this category, much as it has been difficult to identify language impairment as a whole (Stark and Tallal, 1981).

One of the most significant contributions to the arguments in favour of a specific deficit has been made by Tallal and her colleagues (Tallal *et al.*, 1980). In a series of articles they showed that language impaired children, between five and nine years of age, scored consistently more poorly than same-age controls, when asked to discriminate auditory stimuli. Furthermore, performance was affected both by the duration of the tone administered and by the length of the interval between tones. They explained this in terms of the children having a specific difficulty perceiving rapidly occurring acoustic events. This, they argued, provided conclusive evidence that there was a specific deficit peculiar to s.l.i. children.

In fact, the argument for a specific disorder of this type is now being called into question (Leonard, 1987). Tomblin and Quine

(1983), for example, have suggested that the auditory discrimination skill identified by Tallal and her colleagues can be taught in a way that other aspects of language can be taught. They conclude that language learning and speed of acoustic recall are skills which develop alongside one another rather than in sequence. The fact that the controls in the Tallal studies were of the same age as the study group children, rather than matched for language, may mean that the language level of the children concerned may have adversely affected the capacity to recall auditory stimuli. It is also difficult to know what these results mean in terms of the preschool population who would not be expected to have this level of awareness about the process of language. Finally, it is not clear what the exact relationship between these skills and language might be.

It has become increasingly clear that language skills are also related to other symbolic skills. The best example of this is play. It has been shown by a number of commentators that children with poor language development also have difficulty playing. Brown *et al.* (1975) showed that specific language impaired children were less adaptive in their use of objects than a group of age-matched controls. In this case the children, aged three to five years, were given a set of objects and asked to pretend they were at a birthday party. Williams (1978) specifically counted the number of symbolic acts in a play session and found that language impaired children aged 2 years 6 months to 5 years 6 months performed significantly less well than age-matched controls. Terrell *et al.* (1984) used a specific measure of play and compared language impaired children (aged 2 years 8 months to 4 years 1 month) to one group of children controlled for language level and a second for age. The results indicated that the language impaired children performed at a higher level than the children with equivalent language ages, but lower than the children matched for age. Poor play skills are also found in children with broader developmental difficulties but the fact that the low-level symbolic skills of language impaired children do not compare with their other non-verbal skills suggests that the underlying difficult may be specific to symbolization rather than to language.

Another interesting aspect of language impairment referred to by Leonard (1987) is that of mental imagery. Inhelder (1963) first noted that a child (aged 9 years 6 months) with specific language impairment also seemed to experience a specific difficulty describing the relative positions of a tilted jug and the surface of the water within that jug. Kamhi (1981) compared a group of language impaired children with one matched for mental age and a second matched for mean length of utterance on a variety of Piagetian tasks. The language impaired group only stood out at one task – one in which children were required to feel the shape of a geometric figure and then select the corresponding form from a visual array. Interestingly, the language impaired group again performed better than their language-matched controls. The task in question was the only one specifically involving imaging and the results led the authors to conclude that it was the ability to hold a visual representation of the task which was lacking. Camarata *et al.*, (1981) took age matched and mean length of utterance (m.l.u.) matched controls and compared their response to a task which required the children to appreciate perspective of a given set of objects from the angle of the presenter. Once again, the language impaired children performed much less well than their age matched peers but better than the younger children with equivalent language scores.

It does seem that there are a variety of tasks which are not essentially linguistic but which language impaired children nevertheless find particularly difficult. Despite this, the term s.l.i. is generally retained because it suggests a broad category of children who, when assessed on standardized tests, perform disproportionately poorly on language subtests. Inevitably this depends on the measure used. Thus if the test is largely perceptual, such as the Leiter (Johnston 1982), then these children are much less likely to present with cognitive problems. But if the test requires linguistic elicitation, albeit of non-verbal tasks, the results may be confounded by the child's linguistic difficulties.

Despite these uncertainties as to how specific 'specific language impairment' is, the term continues to be widely used by many of those working with these children. Children are assessed in the UK and admitted to language units on the basis of this distinction between language difficulties which are associated with general developmental delay and those which are specific to language. Similarly these children are enrolled into programmes in the US on the basis of this type of distinction. Inevitably, disagreements as to the most valid provision accompany such decisions. The distinction continues to have a clinical value which may not be wholly supported by the literature.

THE DELAY/DISORDER DISTINCTION

One feature of the early development of language which any classification system must take into account is the fact that a substantial proportion of children who are slow in starting to speak subsequently go on to develop language perfectly normally. To provide for this 'developmental noise', a further stratum of nomenclature has developed. Children are said to be suffering from **language disorder** or **language delay**. The two terms are supposed to refer to distinct clinical groups. Traditionally the former comprise a group for whom the pattern of language development has been disturbed and for whom the prognosis is poor. The latter comprises a group of children who develop language normally but at a slower rate than their peers and for whom the prognosis is considered good.

However when the distinction is examined in more detail, it is not always used consistently. Thus 'disorder' may refer to

1. a disorder within the various components of language – thus with a more pronounced problem in phonology than syntax. This is the type of approach suggested by Bishop and Edmundson (1987a). For them, it is the pattern of skills which is the best determinant of outcome.
2. a disorder between the language function and other cognitive functions.
3. a disorder in which the development of syntax or phonology is out of synchronization with the other elements of that system. Thus prepositions or velar plosives (/k g/) might be said to be expected at one level but only develop much later, long after the other elements appropriate for the same level have already developed. Despite early optimism that this may be the case, Morehead and Ingram (1973) found that language-disordered children developed their early syntax in much the same order as normal children. The evidence from Bates *et al.* (1988) suggests that care needs to be taken in assuming that order, at least with the very young child, constitutes a problem in itself.

Similarly 'delay' refers to

1. an overall delay of the components of language in relation to all other skills, for example such that the child's language presents as that of a three-year-old at chronological age five. The child then catches up once the appropriate

stimulation is provided, so that no distinction can be made between the child and his peers.

2. the same as 1) above but with no commitment to the concept of catching up. Thus it would be possible to speak of a ten-year-old with a language delay.

The difficulty has arisen largely because the terms have often been used in an imprecise fashion. And this is not surprising, once we try to identify the conditions for a child to be in one group or another. Of course it might be possible to make the distinction retrospectively. But this is not very helpful from a clinical perspective. Furthermore it poses problems for therapists or teachers attempting to show that their treatment is effective. If the child improves it might be argued that he can only have been delayed and so the problem would have resolved spontaneously.

The term 'delay' suggests that older children would present in a similar manner to younger children with equivalent language levels. But this is rarely the case. The life experiences of the older child make it highly unlikely that the communication performance of the two children will be comparable.

Case Study 2.1

Joanne was 4½ when she was first identified by her nursery teacher as having difficulties with her speech. She had started at the nursery six months before, having just moved into the area. She had been to a playgroup before this. A referral to the speech therapist indicated that she had marked phonological problems. She consistently substituted alveolar sounds (t/ d) for velars (/k g/) and fricatives (f/ʃ/s). When assessed on a standardized language test she presented as having comprehension within normal limits but with a delay in her expressive language of two years. However, when looking at Joanne in her nursery, it was clear the implications of her communication problem went beyond her speech. She played on her own, often repetitively following simple routines with dolls. She would sit looking at books and her attention was generally good. The books that she would look at would be the same as those chosen by her peers but she would refuse to try and retell the story in more than single words. Unlike most of her peers, she showed no willingness to respond to the printed word. Furthermore she found it difficult to relate to adults, either avoiding them altogether or clinging to those that were most familiar.

Comment: Joanne was clearly delayed in that her expressive language was similar to that of a younger child. But she had developed a range of associated behaviours which indicated that she was avoiding aspects of communication which required use of those language skills. This in turn dramatically affected her use of language such that she presented neither as a 2½-year-old nor a 4½-year-old.

Attempts at unravelling the two categories have, to date, proved rather unsatisfactory. For this reason, the term 'language impairment' is adopted in the present volume because it suggests the severity of the problem without forcing a rather unhappy distinction between delay and disorder. It is recognized that there will be subcategorizations within this group of the type discussed in the previous chapter, but that prognosis in each case will be dependent on a variety of factors such as the pervasive nature of the impairment, the degree of impairment of the subcategory concerned and, finally, a range of mitigating circumstances which interact with the skills of the child – the temperament of the child, the home environment, the school environment, the effects of therapeutic intervention or the outcome of medical treatment. These categories have yet to be adequately developed. Furthermore, the use of the single term 'impairment' suggests that, albeit at quite a gross level, there is a degree of homogeneity in the group of children concerned. In other words they are all impaired to the extent that they all have recognizable difficulties in their communication.

PERSISTENCE

Implicit in the need to identify language impaired children at an early stage is the understanding that the problems which they experience are not simply transitory. If the problems do not persist and children invariably 'grow out of it', there would be little point in trying to affect their course through intervention. So it is necessary to examine these children prospectively.

Early follow-up studies of children in specific units for the language impaired have indicated that many children continue to have difficulties well after leaving the unit concerned. Griffiths (1969) and Garvey and Gordon (1973), Weiner (1972, 1974) and

Aram, Ekelman and Nation (1984) all indicate that such children go on to have a poor prognosis in terms of all aspects of their performance, i.e. reading, writing, social adjustment etc. These studies were dealing with children who were clearly experiencing the most severe of problems and may not be representative of the language impaired population which would include a great many with milder presentations. For this reason it is important to look at studies that have examined populations which are more representative.

The same general pattern emerges. Richman *et al.* (1982) found that three-year-olds with poor language development had a consistently poor outcome at eight years. This poor performance extended beyond speech and language to behaviour problems, poor reading skills and low overall IQ. This last point is particularly interesting because their language impaired group was identified as expressively impaired. Silva, Williams and McGee (1987) found that when children of the same initial age were followed up at eleven years, those with early language problems were also likely to experience low IQ scores, poor progress in reading and writing and behaviour problems.

Bishop and Edmundson (1987a) have provided some contradictory evidence which needs to be considered. They followed up a group of language impaired children between the ages of four and 5½ and found that their language development increased at the same rate as the normal children who were used as controls. The authors suggested that this should be considered evidence that these children do catch up in the end. Any variation in the speed at which children catch up will be determined by the interaction between the various components of language. They found a single measure of sequencing ability to be the best predictor of language performance at 5½ years. In other words there are salient aspects of communicative ability which may serve as indicators. One of the models which they suggest consists of a set of mountains which are submerged or exposed depending on the water level. Each mountain corresponds to an impairment in an area of functioning and is represented in Figure 2.1. The more a mountain is exposed the more severe the impairment, and the higher the mountain the more vulnerable the function. Thus the severity of the impairment is analogous with water level. As the children improve the pattern changes to one higher in the series.

From the perspective of early identification it would therefore follow that children with phonological problems alone would have a better prognosis and would, therefore, not be a target while those with a combination of semantic and syntactic problems would be. The children in the Bishop and Edmundson study (Bishop and Adams, 1990) have been followed up through to eight years and reassessed for their language and reading skills. The results indicate that those children who had pervasive language difficulties at 5½ continued to have poor oral language and were experiencing difficulties with their literacy skills at eight. As predicted by the model in Figure 2.1 the authors found only a weak association between phonological development at the younger age and subsequent reading performance. Yet this issue has still to be satisfactorily resolved. Shriburg and Kwiatowski (1988) followed up a number of children with phonological disorders alone and found that their problems persisted into the school years and detrimentally affected reading and writing performance.

These results suggest that a large proportion of children who have difficulties with language in the preschool years go on to have persistent problems. It may be that those problems initially presenting in the form of language impairment go on to 'translate'

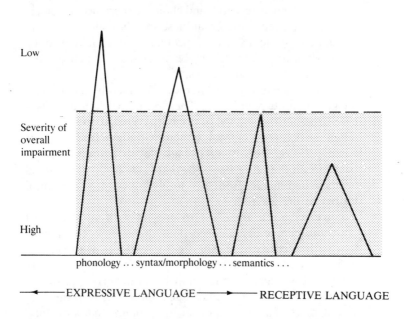

phonology ... syntax/morphology ... semantics ...

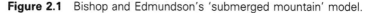

Figure 2.1 Bishop and Edmundson's 'submerged mountain' model.

into other areas of development, and that language itself does improve to a reasonable level with time. Clearly, as a population, the language impaired group is at risk in the long term.

SUMMARY AND CONCLUSIONS

The following points may be extracted from the preceding discussion

- Attempts at rationalizing the prevalence data suggest three bands. In reality the distinctions between these bands are likely to prove artificial. The subject is fraught with problems of operational definitions.
- Terminology in the area has often confused rather than simplified the issues concerned. Given the number of disciplines contributing to the discussion of these children, this is hardly surprising.
- It is suggested that the term **language impairment** be used as a first level description and that under it there should be a series of specific conditions which become increasingly well delineated as research and clinical experience develops. Although it is recognized that these specific conditions make up a heterogeneous set of problems, it should also be acknowledged that there may be an underlying neurodevelopmental delay in many cases.
- There are essentially two methods for identifying the language impaired population. The first is to adopt a statistically predetermined level of disability. The second relies on adopting accepted clinical symptomatology. Both present complications; the former because levels adopted rely on convention, the latter because what is clinically determined needs to be reliable. Both are closely linked into the natural history of the disorder.
- Younger children are likely to present with more general difficulties than older children. This almost inevitably means that early identification will pick up children with general difficulties which only subsequently become more clearly defined. This suggests that it may be a red herring to search for only the most specific language impairments in the preschool years. This is supported by evidence that s.l.i. may not be as specific as originally thought.

- One of the most pervasive problems from the point of view of the clinician is to discriminate between the children who are likely to go on to have schooling difficulties and those who will have 'caught up' by the time they have reached school. It may be that it is the degree of difficulty in any one linguistic modality which is the determining factor. Equally it may be that there is a particularly disadvantageous combination of linguistic skills which could be used to predict which children should be picked out. A third option is that there may be an interaction between non-linguistic factors and the child's language skills, resulting in a cumulative educational disadvantage. And it is to these associated non-linguistic factors that we turn next.

REFERENCES

American Psychiatric Association (1980) *Diagnostic and Statistical Manual of Mental Disorders*, 3rd Edn, APA, Washington D.C.

Aram, D. E. and Nation, J. E. (1975) Patterns of language behaviour in children with developmental language disorders. *Journal of Speech and Hearing Research*, **18**, 229–241.

Aram, D. E., Ekelman, B. L. and Nation, J. E. (1984) Preschoolers with language disorders: ten years later. *Journal of Speech and Hearing Research*, **27**, 232–244.

Barker, D. J. P. and Rose, G. (1984) *Epidemiology in Medical Practice*, Churchill Livingstone, Edinburgh.

Bates, E., Bretherton, I. and Snyder, L. (1988) *From First Words to Grammar*, Cambridge University Press, Cambridge.

Bax, M., Hart, H. and Jenkins, S. (1980) Assessment of speech and language development in the young child. *Pediatrics*, **66**, 350–354.

Bax, M., Hart, H. and Jenkins, S. (1983) The behaviour, development and health of the young child: implications for care. *British Medical Journal*, **286**, 1793–1796.

Beitchman, J. H. (1985) Speech and language impairment and psychiatric risk – towards a model of neurodevelopmental immaturity. *Psychiatric Clinics of North America*, **8**, 721–725.

Beitchman, J. H., Nair, R., Clegg, M. *et al.* (1986) Prevalence of speech and language disorders in 5-year-old kindergarten children in the Ottawa Careton Region. *Journal of Speech and Language Disorders*, **51**, 98–110.

Bishop, D. and Adams, C. (1990) A prospective study of the relationship between specific language impairment, phonological disorders and reading retardation. *Journal of Child Psychology and Psychiatry*, **31** (7), 1027–1051.

Bishop, D. and Edmundson, A. (1987a) Language impaired 4-year-olds: Distinguishing transient from persistent impairment. *Journal of Speech and Hearing Disorders*, **52**, 156–173.

Bishop, D. and Edmundson, A. (1987b) Specific language impairment as a maturational lag: Evidence from longitudinal data on language and motor development. *Development Medicine and Child Neurology*, **29**, 442–459.

Bishop, D. and Rosenbloom, L. (1987) Classification of childhood language disorders, in *Language Development and Disorders* (78) (eds. W. Yule and M. Rutter), MacKeitt Press, Oxford, pp. 16–41.

Brown, J., Redmond, A., Bass, K. *et al.* (1975) Symbolic play in normal and language impaired children. Paper presented at the American Speech-Language-Hearing Association Convention Washington D.C.

Camarata, S., Newhall, M. and Rugg, B. (1981) Perspective taking in normal and language disordered children. *Proceedings from the Symposium on Research in Child Language Disorder*, **2**, 81–88.

Crystal, D. (1981) *Clinical Linguistics*, Springer-Verlag, New York.

Fundudis, T., Kolvin, I. and Garside, R. (1979) *Speech Retarded and Deaf Children: their Psychological Development*, Academic Press, London.

Garvey, M. and Gordon, N. (1973) A follow up study of children with disorders of speech development. *British Journal of Disorders of Human Communication*, **8**, 17–26.

Griffiths, C. (1969) A follow up study of children with disorders of speech. *British Journal of Disorders of Communication*, **4**, 446–456.

Ingram, T. (1963) Report of the dysphasia subcommittee of the Scottish Paediatric Association. Unpublished paper quoted in Randall, D., Reynell R., and Curwen, M. (1974).

Ingram, T. (1972) The classification of speech and language disorders in young children, in *The Child with Delayed Speech*, (eds M. Rutter and J. Martin), Heinemann, London.

Inhelder, B. (1963) Observations sur les aspects operatifs et figuratifs de la pensee chez des infants dysphasiques. *Problemes de Psycholinguistique*, **6**, 143–153.

Johnston, J. (1982) Interpreting the Leiter IQ: Performance profiles of young normal and language disordered children. *Journal of Speech and Hearing Research*, **25**, 291–296.

Kamhi, A. (1981) Nonlinguistic symbolic and conceptual abilities of language impaired and normally developing children. *Journal of Speech and Hearing Research*, **24**, 446–453.

Lahey, M. (1988) *Language Disorders and Language Development*, Macmillan, London.

Leonard, L. (1987) Is specific language impairment a useful construct? In *Advances in Applied Psycholinguistics*, Volume 1, (ed. S. Rosenberg), Erlbaum, Hillsdale, N.J., pp. 1–39.

Morehead, D. and Ingram, D. (1973) The development of base syntax in normal and linguistically deviant children. *Journal of Speech and Hearing Disroders*, **16**, 330–352.

Morley, M. (1957) *The Development and Disorders of Speech in Childhood*, Livingstone, London.

Randall, D., Reynell, J. and Curwen, M. (1974) A study of language development in a sample of three-year-olds. *British Journal of Disorders of Communication*, **9**, 3–16.

Rapin, I. and Allen, D. A. (1987) Developmental dysphasia and autism in preschool children: characteristics and subtypes, in *Proceedings of the First International Symposium of Specific Speech and Language Disorders in Children*, Association For All Speech Impaired Children, Middlesex.

Reynell, J. and Huntley, M. (1985) *The Reynell Developmental Language Scales*, NFER: Nelson, Windsor.

Richman, N., Stevenson, J. and Graham, P. (1982) *Preschool to School: A Behavioural Study*, Academic Press, London.

Rutter, M., Tizard, J. and Whitmore, K. (1970) *Education Health and Behaviour*, Longmans, London.

Silva, P. A., McGee, R. and Williams, S. (1983) Developmental language delay from three to seven years and its significance for low intelligence and reading difficulties at age seven. *Developmental Medicine and Child Neurology*, **25**, 783–793.

Silva, P. A., Williams, S. and McGee, R. (1987) A longitudinal study of children with developmental language delay at age three: later intelligence, reading and behaviour problems. *Developmental Medicine and Child Neurology*, **29**, 630–640.

Snyder-McClean, L. and McClean, J. E. (1987) Effectiveness of early intervention for children with language and communication disorders, in *The Effectiveness of Early Intervention for At-Risk and Handicapped Children*, (eds M. J. Guralnick and F. C. Bennett), Academic Press, Orlando, Florida, pp. 213–271.

Stark, R. and Tallal, P. (1981) Selection of children with specific language deficits. *Journal of Speech and Hearing Disorders*, **46**, 114–122.

Shriberg, L. and Kwiatowski, J. (1988) A follow-up study of children with phonological disorders of unknown origin. *Journal of Speech and Hearing Disorders*, **53**, 144–53.

Tallal, P., Stark, R., Kallman, C. and Mellits, D. (1980) Developmental dysphasia: The relationship between acoustic processing deficits and verbal processing. *Neuropsychologia*, **18**, 273–284.

Terrell, B., Schwarz, R. Prelock, P. and Messick, C. (1984) Symbolic play in normal and language impaired children. *Journal of Speech and Hearing Research*, **27**, 424–429.

Tomblin, J. B. and Quine, M. (1983) The contribution of perceptual learning to performance on the repetition task. *Journal of Speech and Hearing Research*, **26**, 369–372.

Weiner, P. (1972) The preceptual level functioning of dysphasic children: A follow up study. *Journal of Speech and Hearing Disorders*, **165**, 423–438.

Weiner, P. (1974) A language delayed child in adolescence. *Journal of Speech and Hearing Disorders*, **36**, 202–212.

Wells, G. (1985) *Language Development in the Preschool Years*, Cambridge University Press, Cambridge.

Wells, G. (1986) Variation in child language, in *Language Acquisition*, (eds P. Fletcher and M. Garman), Cambridge University Press, Cambridge.

Williams, R. (1978) Play behaviour of language-handicapped and normal speaking preschool children. Paper presented at the American Speech-Language-Hearing Association Convention San Francisco.

3

Factors associated with language impairment

James Law

In the last chapter we saw how early attempts at defining language impairment have proved to be more successful in theory than in practice. Despite various attempts to provide a complete classificatory system, we are still at the stage of describing the conditions themselves. This chapter expands this descriptive framework to include factors found to be associated with language impairment which are not linguistic in nature. In some cases these are known to cause language difficulties. More commonly they co-occur and the nature of the relationship between them remains unclear.

GENDER

The relationship between gender and language development may be viewed from two perspectives. The first refers to the normal population, the second to the language impaired population. The most coherent résumé of the literature on the effects of gender on language has been made by Maccoby and Jacklin (1975). Where differences do exist they tend to favour girls, especially in underprivileged populations (Schachter *et al.*, 1978). The conventional interpretation for this is that boys develop more slowly, and thereby have a greater vulnerability to hazards of all sorts (Yule and Rutter, 1987). Yet Bee and her colleagues (Bee *et al.*, 1984) maintain that rather than a greater sensitivity in all aspects of development, there are particular experiences which produce different effects for boys than for girls. Thus they found that boys' language development was more related to the mother's developmental expectations, the extent of the father's involvement in the infant's early care, the provision of appropriate play materials and the extent of parental life change.

The alternative approach is to study the clinical population of language impaired children. The figures for the ratio of boys to girls with specific language impairment are quite consistent, ranging as they do between two and three to one (Morley, 1972; Silva, 1989). Fundudis *et al.* (1979) quote a ratio of 1.7:1 for a total speech retarded group, further dividing this into 2:1 for a residual speech retarded group, and 1:1 for a pathologically deviant group. Drillien and Drummond (1983) quote a slightly higher proportion of 2.5:1 for children with a principal diagnosis of speech disorder. Robinson, reporting on ten different studies, reports an average of 2.82:1 (Robinson, 1987). In a more specific example, Aram and Nation (1982) report a ratio of 2.9:1 for children with verbal apraxia.

MEDICAL FACTORS

Similarly there are two methods which can be used for studying the relationship between language and medical history. The first involves studying sick children or those who are medically 'at risk'. The second comes from examining a population of children with language impairment for evidence of adverse medical histories.

The case for the former is not now disputed. A number of studies have shown that children who are premature, of low birth weight and who are small for dates (Rocissano and Yatchmink, 1983; Largo *et al.*, 1986), are all at risk of subsequent problems of which communication is likely to be a part. In a study of low birth weight children (less than 100 g.), Grunau *et al.* (1990) have shown that the children had less complex expression and lower receptive understanding, auditory memory and verbal reasoning at three years. Language outcome was related to specific dysfunctions rather than global measures of postnatal illness. Low birthweight and 'small for dates' children seem to find the whole process of interaction harder to master than their normal peers and this in turn makes it harder for their parents to interact with them effectively. 'Failure to thrive' children for whom oromotor dysfunction was a consistent feature have been shown to have feeding problems which are in turn related to parent/child interaction and ultimately expressive language difficulties (Mathieson *et al.*, 1989). There is also extensive evidence that most chromosomal conditions which affect cognitive development also affect language (Sparks, 1984). In some cases, for example children with Down's syndrome, the children have problems with their expressive language, above and beyond their cognitive skills (Cardoso-Martins *et al.*, 1985).

Evidence from the second perspective is less forthcoming. If you study more severe cases of children with language impairment you are likely to find chromosomal abnormalities. Indeed Robinson (1987) found 3–5% of children in a school for the most severe cases of speech and language disorder to have such abnomality. Butler *et al.* (1973) found a high percentage of children presenting with speech problems at age seven to have been preterm. Similarly Lassman *et al.* (1980) found maternal age of less than 18 years, higher parity, maternal height of less than 60 inches, very low or very high weight gain during pregnancy, all to be unfavourably associated with subsequent speech and language performance. Interestingly enough, no relationship was established between method of delivery and outcome. Apgar score was only relevant in that scores of 0–3 were subsequently related to hearing-test results. Similarly a proportion of those with marked language problems will also have experienced epilepsy. In short genetic defects and those associated with cerebral trauma are likely to be directly responsible for language difficulties, while factors associated with the medical environment are only likely to contribute to language impairment if they are sufficiently severe to cause more general difficulties.

In recent years increased attention has been paid to neurodevelopmental or maturational lags experienced by language impaired children. Beitchman (1985) has suggested that evidence from the psychiatric examination of language impaired children supports a neurodevelopmental association. Similarly Bishop and Edmundson (1987) found that language impaired children had particular difficulty with a peg-moving task. The language difficulty was closely associated with slow motor performance with both hands. Furthermore those children for whom the language impairment resolved between four and 5½ also improved in their manual skills. Using this model, outcome for the s.l.i. child is predicted on the basis of the severity of the neurodevelopmental lag. Such findings are clearly in line with those presented in Chapter 2 relating to specific language impairment. It would appear that although these children have significant language problems in the absence of global cognitive difficulties of the type identified by standardized assessments of intelligence, they often present with comparatively subtle neurodevelopmental problems.

IMPAIRED SENSORY INPUT

Sensory input, for the purposes of the present discussion, is confined to hearing and vision. Children with visual impairment achieve language milestones at or near the ages expected for sighted children. Yet differences have been observed in the use and the nature of the language which is acquired. For example, a number of authors have noted a tendency of blind children to have particular difficulties with the I/you pronoun distinction (Freeman and Blockberger, 1987). These children are likely to have problems with both representational play and in all aspects of non-verbal communication. It is important that, to affect language development, visual difficulties have to be severe. There is, of course, no reason why language impaired children should be any more prone to visual difficulties.

Hearing will be discussed at length in Chapter 5. For the present it is sufficient to say that children with 'sensori-neural' hearing losses affecting the neurological components of the hearing apparatus are clearly at risk for marked language problems. Conductive hearing loss, which affects the transfer of sound to the organs of the ear, is much more common in young children. One of the most common causes of conductive hearing loss is ear infection associated with colds which are, in turn, the most common of all childhood ailments. While it is now clear that children with severe hearing loss of this type will have difficulties in communicating, it remains uncertain as to exactly what the relationship is between slight or fluctuating hearing loss and language development. Bax, Hart and Jenkins (1980) found a link between history of ear infection and abnormal speech and language development at two years. Even slight hearing losses need to be monitored carefully and clinicians treating the medical aspects of the problem will need to keep a close eye on the development of language skills. It does not necessarily follow that a child with a language impairment has a hearing loss or vice versa but there is clearly a relationship between the two which cannot be ignored.

In terms of early identification, the child of whom the greatest care needs to be taken is the one with fluctuating conductive hearing loss. Significant sensory losses of both vision and hearing are more likely to be identified by parents and the necessary provision made. By contrast the child with conductive hearing loss may experience persistent problems but remain undetected. The fluctuating loss may appear less severe but the unpredictability which it entails can be very difficult for the young child to cope with.

ENVIRONMENTAL AND SOCIAL FACTORS

Adverse environmental factors have general deleterious consequences and language is simply one part of the equation. For example diet affects cerebral capacity which in turn is likely to affect language development (Crawford *et al.*, 1986). Nevertheless some authors have suggested that there may be specific consequences of lead pollution (Mayfield, 1983) or foetal alcohol syndrome (Shaywitz *et al.*, 1981). As interest in the make-up of the physical environment, food additives, pollution, etc. increase so too will our understanding of the number of possible contributary factors. Such investigations are severely hampered by methodology. And it is often very difficult to know what sense to make of them in clinical terms.

The debate as to whether social class affects language development is one to which considerable attention has already been directed (see Edwards, 1989). While children from lower socioeconomic groups do generally perform more poorly on language assessments than do their middle class counterparts, it is likely that their performance is as much to do with the structure of the tests used and with parental expectation as it is to do with specifically linguistic skills. In general, the crude stratification of social class is not very revealing. Instead researchers have turned to the nature of the environment experienced by the child.

One schedule which has been developed specifically to describe the domestic environment is the Home Observation for Measurement of the Environment (HOME) (Bradley and Caldwell, 1977). It consists of 45 items assessing six categories of stimulation available to the infant. These are

1. Emotional and verbal responsivity of the mother.
2. Avoidance of restriction and punishment.
3. Organization of the physical and temporal environment.
4. Provision of appropriate play materials.
5. Maternal involvement with the child.
6. Opportunities for variety in daily activities.

The schedule has been used in a variety of circumstances. One of the most extensive studies is reported by Bee *et al.* (1982). The authors used the HOME on the 193 children in their study following them through from 4 to 48 months assessing IQ and language skills at a number of points. They found the following three factors to be the best predictors of performance.

1. Mother–child interaction.
2. Environmental quality (the HOME).
3. Mother's education and the support available to her within the family.

The authors concluded that it was possible to use the HOME to predict both IQ and language skill at all the ages tested. The problem, of course, with this type of study is that it deals with an ostensibly normal population and it is not necessarily possible to extrapolate the results by saying that language impairment is a function of social factors *per se*.

Fundudis *et al.* (1979) point out that environmental factors do clearly influence children's verbal abilities. In their study, two distinct groups were identified. The first, known as the 'pathologically deviant group', comprised handicapped children while their 'residual speech retarded group' had language problems in the absence of other handicapping conditions. They showed that there was increased evidence of stress and tension within the families of both groups. There was a greater number of marital separations and an increase in maternal psychological stress in their speech retarded groups. The authors attributed the social stress to the child's handicap in the first group but maintained that the problems in the latter group were 'more a reflection of tensions associated with greater loadings of social factors' (p. 43).

It seems likely that very poor circumstances, or a combination of a number of adverse factors, may have detrimental effects. But beyond this one has to be very cautious about simply associating poor development with socio-economic status. The fact is that children have repeatedly proved to be astonishingly robust in their response to such disadvantage (Clarke and Clarke, 1976). So it seems highly unlikely that in most cases adverse social circumstances are responsible for more than comparatively slight variation in language development (Puckering and Rutter, 1987). Even when disadvantage does seem to be the primary reason, it is insufficient to explain all the variability that does occur (Mogford and Bishop, 1988).

FAMILIAL FACTORS

Position within the family is often considered to be a relevant social factor. There is a tendency for younger children from larger families to have lower intellectual ability and to be lower achievers in school (Butler *et al.*, 1973; Rutter and Madge, 1976). It remains to be seen how far results for overall intellectual achievement may be generalized to language development. It is commonly assumed that the first-born child has more direct verbal input from the parents while second-born and later children have to rely on their siblings for input. While this may be true in many families, care must be taken in assuming that it always holds true. In certain circumstances first-born children can have a more disruptive effect on a new parent and this may result in rejection. Parents are likely to feel more confident in their handling of the second-born child.

If there is little evidence that factors directly associated with socio-economic status create language impairment as such, the same can not now be said to be true of family history. A recent study (Tallal *et al.*, 1989) has shown that families of specifically language impaired children had a significantly higher proportion of first-degree relatives than families with matched controls. This undoubtedly lends weight to the inclusion of such a characteristic in any clinical judgement. Whether this is a function of some inherited characteristic which specifically relates to language or whether the language input that the child receives is detrimentally affected by a persistently poor adult model is not clear. Recently some evidence has emerged that, in the case of developmental dyspraxia at least, there may be a specific autosomal recessive trait which affects a considerable proportion of familial members (Hurst *et al.*, 1990).

It is difficult to be sure that parental report of a difficulty would necessarily correspond to an impairment in current clinical terms. Alongside the hazards of retrospective judgement is the fact that such problems have only been described comparatively recently. There may simply not have been the services available in the preceding generation to make the necessary identification possible. It is quite possible that the association is stronger than it already appears.

PARENT/CHILD INTERACTION

It would seem to be intuitively likely that the child's language development will be affected by the way that he or she is spoken to. Yet the literature suggests that the relationship between parental input and the child's output is not necessarily a simple case of the former creating the latter. Indeed the discussion in

Chapter 1 shows quite clearly the agentive role which the very young child plays in the interaction process.

There are three main sources of evidence which shed light on the relationship.

1. Cases of extreme deprivation.
2. Evidence for a distinct parenting speech style or 'motherese'.
3. Evidence from the population of language impaired children.

Cases of extreme deprivation

There have now been a number of well-documented cases of children who have been severely neglected (see Skuse, 1988, for a review). When they have been discovered these children invariably have severe communication problems. Fortunately these more extreme cases are comparatively rare. Yet there is now evidence that children who have been abused and emotionally neglected as infants may also be at risk of language difficulties (Law and Conway, 1991). Such evidence as there is indicates that even in the most severe cases it is possible to intervene by changing the child's environment, which in turn readily affects the child's language abilities. The child who has experienced neglect may be most at risk for persistent problems simply because the condition may not be considered sufficiently serious to warrant the kind of environment change which might improve the course of language development.

Evidence for a distinct parenting speech style or 'motherese'

We have seen in Chapter 1 that one of the hallmarks of the baby's first year of life is the interaction between parent and child. So robust is the infant's desire to communicate that it sometimes seems as if it is impossible to stop language from developing. Indeed the original impetus for the study of maternal speech style came from Chomsky's (1957) assumption that children learn language in spite of the apparently corrupt and ungrammatical speech that parents use to their children. He used this argument as a justification for his claim that children have an inate capacity to learn language which is not subject to environmental factors. Taken to its logical conclusion this argument assumes that children will learn language irrespective of the quality of their linguistic environment.

Brown, in his seminal work *A First Language: The Early Stages* (1973), refuted Chomsky's claim that the parent's speech style was inadequate as a model from which to learn language. Rather he concluded that the mother's speech style to small children differed from that to others in a consistent and predictable fashion. The characteristics which are generally ascribed to 'motherese' are as follows:

1. It is spoken at a slower rate and with more clearly defined pauses than language between adults. It is also in a higher pitch range.
2. The sentence forms tend to be short and grammatical. There will be few grammatically complex structures.
3. It is very repetitive both of the adult and the child utterance. Where changes do occur they tend to be in recasting of the child's previous utterances.
4. The vocabulary used refers to objects and people immediately experienced by the child. Consequently it is limited and concrete rather than abstract.
5. The adult shows an awareness of the child's level and seems to unconsciously promote the child's linguistic development by using structures slightly more advanced than those used by the child. Thus to the 'miaow' of the 14-month-old the mother might say 'yes, it's a cat' while to the 2½-year-old's 'dinner gone' she might say 'yes, you've eaten up all your dinner'.

Although these characteristics have been widely accepted there has been some considerable discussion as to their function (Wanner and Gleitman, 1986). It seems unlikely that quality of parental input does more than influence style of infant output. Motherese, in itself, should not be seen as causing language development. As Snow (1986) has observed, the 'semantic contingency' identified in North American and English cultures is not necessarily universal. There is no evidence that societies which do not encourage this style of parent/child interaction learn language any more slowly than those that do.

Evidence from the population of language impaired children

Wulbert *et al.* (1975) found that the parents of language impaired children were much less responsive and much more critical than the parents of children with normally developing language. Mothers of the language impaired children met the physical needs of their children but 'lived together in a parallel fashion' with their children rather than actively interacting with them.

More recently (Conti-Ramsden and Friel Patti, 1983; Cunningham *et al.*, 1985) it has been found that language impaired children initiated conversation less than other children which then compelled their mothers to initiate proportionally more than mothers of normally developing children. This in turn had the effect of distorting other aspects of interaction. But these authors did not confirm the finding of Wulbert *et al.* (1975) that the parents were more controlling. Instead they suggest that the language impaired children are inherently more difficult to 'tune in' to.

It is, then, possible to say that the interaction between parent and child will be affected in cases of language impairment. Care needs to be taken in assuming directionality in the distortion of the interaction. Clearly most children learn language perfectly adequately with a minimum of conscious stimulation from their carers. Equally clearly children are unlikely to learn language in a normal fashion when exposed to extremes of sensory deprivation. The evidence suggests that the distortion of interaction which follows in less pronounced cases may well be more as a result of the needs of the child and the difficulty experienced by the parent in attempting to respond to those needs rather than any particular speech style that the parent may use.

BEHAVIOURAL AND PSYCHIATRIC FACTORS

The nature of the relationship between language problems and behavioural difficulties is discussed at length in Chapter 4. Cantwell, Baker and Mathieson (1980) looked at the psychiatric characteristics of a population of 250 children referred to a speech and language clinic in Los Angeles. They found that 53% had a psychiatric diagnosis. The most common of these was attention deficit disorder either with or without hyperactivity.

In a more recent paper the same authors reported on a larger study (Cantwell and Baker, 1987). Six hundred children referred for communication problems were given a psychiatric evaluation. Three clinical groups were identified notably 'pure speech disorders', 'speech and language disorders' and 'pure language disorders'. These three groups were then compared in terms of their psychiatric diagnosis. The two groups with a language component to their disorder had a generally higher rate of psychiatric disorder. Thus 58% of the speech and language disordered group and 73% of the language disordered group were found to have recognizable clinical symptoms. These findings have been corroborated by Beitchman *et al.* (1986) who found 48.7% of a large group of language impaired children with psychiatric problems. Interestingly enough this figure was lower on parental report (22.1%) than on the formal psychiatric examination. This gives clear evidence that the population is at risk of psychiatric problems.

An interesting extension of this approach is to identify subgroups of language problems and look for different patterns of behaviour. In clinical terms it is sometimes assumed that children with comprehension difficulties are more likely to have behaviour problems and the Cantwell and Baker (1987) study referred to above does suggest that it is 'language' rather than speech which is the mediating factor. One study which has particularly addressed this issue is Caulfield *et al.* (1989). These authors looked at a population of very young children presenting with expressive language disorder, and compared them with a group of normally developing children matched for age. They found that these children with expressive problems, but in the absence of developmental delay of comprehension difficulties, still presented with marked behaviour problems. Importantly, the mean age of the children in the study (27.2 months) suggests that such patterns occur at a very early stage in the children's development.

There have been a number of studies which have approached the subject from the other side, looking to establish the proportion of children with behaviour problem who also have language impairment. In their study in Walthamstow, East London, Richman *et al.* (1982) used a non-referred population and found that if they took a definition of behaviour problem which was met by 14% of the population the number of children with significant language problems was 59%. Two studies which have used clinic populations have had not dissimilar results. Gualtieri *et al.* (1983) found 45% of a group of children who were psychiatric in-patients with language problems. At least 28% had deficits below what would be expected for their IQ. Similarly Love and Thompson (1988) looked at the language skills of a sample of children referred to a psychiatric outpatients clinic; 65% of them had a speech or language disorder. These authors also looked at the rate of attention deficit disorder and discovered this to be 73%. Nearly half the children (48%) had a diagnosis of speech and language disorder and attention deficit disorder.

CULTURAL/LINGUISTIC FACTORS

It is sometimes assumed that children who have languages or cultures different from the dominant culture are likely to be at risk of developmental language problems. Although this is essentially not the case there are a number of useful strands which may be teased out which can contribute to our understanding of early identification. Cultures perceive childhood very differently and this may have a dramatic effect on parental expectation of language development. Thus Chasidic Jews see the age of three as being a specific stage through which all children pass but after which expectations change. Boys and girls are for example educated separately from this age (Law and Wallfish, 1991). Harris (1986) has observed that it is assumed in Apache culture that children will not speak to unfamiliar adults. There are many examples of different attitudes to child-rearing in the anthropological literature. It is reasonable to assume that expectations regarding language will vary in a similar way although as yet there is little evidence. It is unclear what this may mean beyond the fact that great care has to be used both when assessing such children and when discussing child development with the parent.

It has been suggested that there is considerable underlying similarity between the structure of widely differing languages (Ferguson and Slobin, 1973). The idea of linguistic universals common to all languages has led to extensive research. Although great similarities have been found it seems likely that there may also be significant differences between languages. Care must always be taken to avoid direct comparison between the language structure of the child with a possible language impairment and the language structure of the language used by the teacher or therapist. It may only be possible to investigate the level of language by means of interpretors or facilitators.

There has been concern expressed that some cultural groups may be referred at a disproportionately high rate. Stewart *et al.* (1986), for example, reported blacks as being overidentified on a series of standardized speech and language assessments. Widerstrom *et al.* (1986) found black children specifically over-represented at three years and 3½ years. This the authors attribute to the children's relative lack of nursery experience. This in turn raises another question and that is the extent to which poor language performance may be a consequence of other factors which are in turn connected to language or cultural group. As we have seen above, social class itself does not look to be closely associated with language impairment, but it is possible that it plays a greater part in contributing to the more conventional sort of delayed language development commonly associated with inadequate stimulation. It seems quite plausible to suggest that the 'stressors' referred to by Bee and her colleagues (Bee *et al.*, 1982) would have precisely this sort of effect.

In some cases there is documented evidence that specific groups experience factors which predetermine children to speech or language problems. There is, for example, evidence that native Americans are predisposed towards otitis media with effusion (Bebout and Mahon, 1987). This being the case it would not be at all surprising to find higher prevalence rates of associated language problems in these populations. Less clearly documented are the effects of immigrant cultures which have to adapt child-rearing practices to a new environment. It is unclear, for example, how well Nigerian families have adapted their extended family systems to urban London (Odebiyi, 1985). There is too little evidence to make any categorical statements regarding the likely prevalence of disorders in different communities. There is a real need for more work in this area. Perhaps one of the greatest obstacles to such work is that there are rarely sufficient resources to carry out adequate studies in the child's country of origin. The other alternative, carrying them out on immigrant populations, is complicated by the linguistic diversity within each group and it is a diversity which changes across time. Furthermore there are often insufficient numbers of any given group to reach any meaningful conclusions.

MULTIVARIATE APPROACHES

The multivariate analysis looks at the extent to which a given set of variables interact to predict a given outcome. It operates on the basis of correlation and so great care should be taken not to confuse the results – i.e. a mathematically derived combination of variables – with a cause. Nevertheless it is worth drawing attention to those attempts that have been made to explain the range of variance of language performance using this technique.

Gold and Berk (1979) studied neurologically impaired children, assessing them for speech and language abilities at three and IQ at four before following them up with an achievement assessment at eight years. The six predictors which the authors used were maternal education, sex, birthweight, infant intelligence, three year speech, hearing and language skills and intelligence at year four. They found that the maximum variance explained by one factor was 16% and by two 20%. Of all the predictors the Stanford Binet at four years was taken to be the best.

The Dunedin Multidisciplinary Child Development Study (Silva and Ferguson, 1980) looked at a sample of 1037 children. As one part of the study a regression analysis was carried out to predict

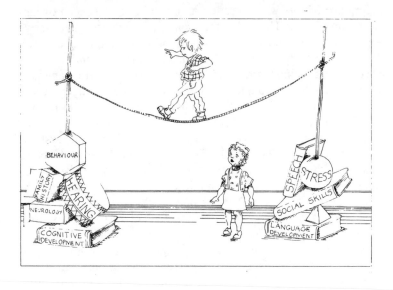

language development at three years. The variables used were maternal general ability, education and training in child development experienced by the mother, socio-economic status, birthweight and 'child experiences'. Once again the model was not very effective in predicting outcome. In this case it succeeded in accounting for only 11% and 7% of variance in the two language measures (comprehension and expression respectively).

In a study referred to earlier in this chapter, Bee and her colleagues (Bee *et al.*, 1982) looked at a wide range of factors including perinatal status, child performance, family characteristics and mother–infant interactions to predict IQ and language skill in a large group of preschool children. The authors concluded that it was possible to explain between 20 and 50% of the variance in IQ or language skill by measuring any of three items, notably the child's early test performance, the mother–infant interaction and the environmental quality as measured on the HOME (Bradley and Caldwell, 1977). Interestingly, given the potential variation in expressive ability identified in Chapter 1, comprehension was consistently better predicted than expression.

In an attempt to distinguish between 51 term and 53 preterm infants in the light of reproductive, perinatal and environmental factors, Siegel (1982) used a similar form of analysis. The children were followed up until they were three years old and assessed on the Stanford Binet and the Reynell Developmental Language Scales. The reproductive variables comprised maternal smoking and the number of previous spontaneous abortions. Perinatal variables included 1 and 5 minutes Apgar scores, hyperbilirubinaemia and, for the preterm infants, gestational age, severity of respiratory distress, birth asphyxia and apnoea. Demographic data included socio-economic status, maternal age, percentage of males born preterm, percentage of first-born preterm. The HOME index (Bradley and Caldwell, 1977) was used on a subsection as a measure of the environment. The combination of reproductive and demographic variables yielded correlations between 0.38 and −0.63. Furthermore the results indicated that it was possible to predict an IQ or a language score at three years of minus one standard deviation or less in 77 to 89% of cases. In all cases the results were more significant for the preterm than the term group.

One study of specific relevance to speech and language impairment was carried out by Schery (1985) in Los Angeles. This study was set up to predict initial presentation and outcome of a special day class for children with severely impaired speech or language. At entry the child's age accounted for 58% of the variance. In other words younger children scored lower initially and improved more than the older children. The other variables accounted for a further 16.5% of the variance, IQ accounting for 2%, socio-economic status for less than 0.5%. The strongest predictor variables included degree of hearing loss, the age the child first walked, the number of childhood accidents and the mother's age at the birth of her child. Measuring performance gain the pre-test scores accounted for 68.4% of the variance while a further 3% was added as a function of the time the children spent on the programme.

These studies show that even with a wide range of variables it is only possible to account for a comparatively small proportion of the variance in language development. The capacity to predict is improved by adding details of the child's earlier performance. The current lack of success in the multivariate model may, as suggested above, be a function of the level of sophistication of the factors included. It may also be a function of the lack of homogeneity of the condition. If the presenting symptoms differ it is no wonder that a single equation will prove inadequate. Multivariate statistics offer us a glimpse of a compositive language impaired child which in reality cannot exist. From the perspective of early identification this is problematical simply because there is unlikely to be any useful record of the child's early language skills. Multivariate approaches are of considerable interest but they are, as yet, unable to approximate the complexities inherent in the process of clinical decision making.

SUMMARY AND CONCLUSIONS

The evidence presented above suggests that language impairment is intricately linked to a whole range of associated factors. In general, the more severe the language difficulty, the stronger the association. Nevertheless we can say that language impairment is more likely to be present if:

1. The child is male.
2. There is a marked adverse medical history, although physical aspects of the medical environment (delivery, etc.) are unlikely to be significant.
3. There is evidence for neurodevelopmental delay.
4. There is evidence of hearing loss. This is clear in cases of pronounced sensori neural or conductive hearing loss. Particular care needs to be taken when examining the relationship between more marginal cases or fluctuating cases of conductive hearing loss.
5. There is a family history of language impairments.
6. There is clear evidence of attachment problems in the first months of life.
7. The child's family experiences a high degree of stress.
8. The child presents with behaviour difficulties.
9. The above occur in combination.

In most cases, a multidimensional model will prove to be more useful than the search for unitary aetiology. It also means that although the process of identifying these children may be complex, a cumulative model is more likely to account for poor outcome than one in which simple linear relationships are examined. Thus a child with intermittent hearing loss will be more at risk if there are attachment difficulties and there is a positive history of lan-

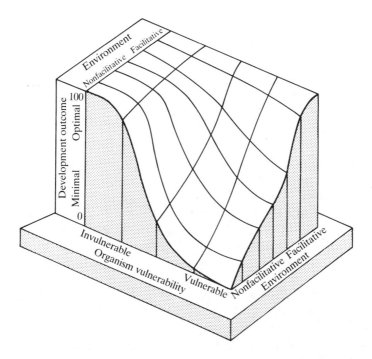

Figure 3.1 Horowitz's model of the interaction between the vulnerability of the child and the quality of the environment. The height of the surface is the 'goodness' of the developmental outcome (like later IQ scores or language skills or social skills). The higher the surface, the better the outcome. As you can see, Horowitz proposes that a vulnerable infant in a nonfacilitative environment will have by far the worst outcome – worse than the simple summing of the effects would predict. (Adapted from Horowitz, 1982.)

guage impairment in the family. The difficulty is that this approach will need to be applied to specific conditions of the type tentatively identified in the previous chapter rather than to the whole population of language impaired children.

This multidimensional approach is well captured by Horowitz (1982) and reported in Bee (1989). Horowitz suggests that the abilities of children can be characterized simultaneously along an internal and an external dimension. The former she terms 'vulnerability' and relates to the child's own capacity to cope with the environment. A child with a hearing loss or a neurodevelopmental lag is clearly at a disadvantage from this point of view. The latter refers to the environment in which the child is raised and the degree of support that is received. Clearly a child who has been neglected will be at risk in this respect. The developmental outcome depends then on an interaction of these two (Figure 3.1). Where the two dimensions are most positive or negative in their interaction there is the most pronounced outcome for better or for worse. While this makes good sense for the purposes of our discussion of language development it remains unclear why those with difficulties in this area should present so differently in clinical terms.

What does this tell us about early identification? Just as we are not looking at a single clinical condition, so we are not looking at a problem which is confined to language. It may be that language is the most pronounced feature of it or perhaps the feature to which our culture is most attuned in educational terms but it is impossible to account for the difficulties purely in linguistic terms. Having said this it is important to recognize that the relationship between these characteristics needs to be weighed up in each case. Just because it is more likely that boys experience language impairment it does not mean that girls are not considered to be at risk at all. Care must be taken not to turn what have been shown to be significant associations into clinical axioms.

Finally, we saw in the previous chapter how many children with early language difficulties go on to have persistent schooling problems. Given the range of associated complications identified here, this is not surprising. The language impaired child may be effectively multiply handicapped. The language may be the most outstanding problem but it is often only the tip of the iceberg.

REFERENCES

Aram, D. and Nation, J. (1982) *Child Language Disorders*, Mosby, St. Louis.

Bax, M., Hart, H. and Jenkins, S. (1980) *The Health Needs of the Pre-School Child*. Unpublished manuscript available from the Community Paediatric Research Unit, Westminster Children's Hospital, Vincent Square, London SW1.

Bebout, J. M. and Mahon, W. J. (1987) Hearing health care and minority populations. *The Hearing Journal*, January, **40**, 7–10.

Bee, H., Bernard, K., Eyres, S. *et al.* (1982) Prediction of IQ and language skills from perinatal status, child performance, family characteristics and mother–infant interaction. *Child Development*, **53**, 1134–1156.

Bee, H., Mitchell, S., Barnard, K. *et al.* (1984) Predicting intellectual outcomes: Sex differences in response to early environmental stimulation. *Sex Roles*, **10**, 783–803.

Bee, H. (1989) *The Developing Child*, 5th edition, Harper and Row, New York.

Beitchman, J. H. (1985) Speech and language impairment and psychiatric risk – towards a model of neurodevelopmental immaturity. *Psychiatric Clinics of North America*, **8**, 721–735.

Beitchman, J. H., Nair, R., Clegg, M. *et al*. (1986) Prevalence of psychiatric disorders in children with speech and language disorders. *Journal of American Academy of Child Psychiatry*, **25** (4), 528–535.

Bishop, D. V. M. and Edmundson, A. (1987) Specific language impairment as a maturational lag: evidence from longitudinal data on language and motor development. *Developmental Medicine and Child Neurology*, **29**, 442–459.

Bradley, R. and Caldwell, B. (1977) Home Observation for Measurement of the Environment: A validation study of screening efficiency. *American Journal of Mental Deficiency*, **81** (5), 417–420.

Brown, R. (1973) *A First Language: The Early Stages*, Penguin, Harmondsworth.

Butler, N., Peckham, C. and Sheridan, M. (1973) Speech defects in children aged 7 years: A national study. *British Medical Journal*, **3**, 253–257.

Cantwell, D. P., Baker, L. and Mathieson, R. (1980) Psychiatric disorders in children with speech and language retardation: Factors associated with development. *Archives of General Psychiatry*, **37**, 423–426.

Cantwell, D. P. and Baker, L. (1987) Prevalence and type of psychiatric disorder and developmental disorder in 3 speech and language groups. *Journal of Communication Disorders*, **20**, 151–160.

Cardoso-Martins, C., Mervis, C. B. and Mervis, C. A. (1985) Early vocabulary acquisition by children with Down's syndrome. *American Journal of Mental Deficiency*, **90**, 177–184.

Caulfield, M. B., Fischel, J. E., DeBaryshe, B. D. and Whitehurst, G. J. (1989) Behavioural correlates of developmental expressive language disorder. *Journal of Abnormal Child Psychology*, **17** (2), 187–201.

Chomsky, N. (1957) *Syntactic Structures*, Mouton, The Hague.

Clarke, A. M. and Clarke, A. D. B. (1976) *Early Experience: Myth and Evidence*, Open Books, London.

Conti-Ramsden, G. and Friel-Patti, S. (1983) Mother's discourse adjustments to language impaired and non language impaired children. *Journal of Speech and Hearing Disorders*, **48**, 360–367.

Crawford, M. A., Doyle, W., Craft, I. L. and Laurence, B. M. (1986) A comparison of food intake during pregnancy and birthweight in high and low socioeconomic groups. *Progress in Lipid Research*, **25**, 249–254.

Cunningham, C., Siegel, L., van de Spuy, H. *et al*. (1985) The behavioural and linguistic interactions of specifically language delayed and normal boys and their mothers. *Child Development*, **56**, 1389–1403.

Drillien, C. and Drummond, M. (1983) *Developmental Screening and the Child with Special Needs*, Heinemann, London.

Edwards, J. (1989) *Language and Disadvantage* (2nd edn), Whurr Publishers, London.

Ferguson, C. A. and Slobin, D. I. (1973) *Studies of Child Language Development*, Holt Rinehart and Winston, New York.

Freeman, R. and Blockberger, S. (1987) Language development and sensory disorder: visual and hearing impairments, in *Language Development and Disorders* (eds W. Yule and M. Rutter), MacKeitt Press, Oxford, pp. 234–247.

Fundudis, T., Kolvin, I. and Garside, R. (1979) *Speech Retarded and Deaf Children: Their Psychological Development*, Academic Press, London.

Gold, P. and Berk, R. (1979) Prediction of the academic success of children with suspected neurological impairment. *Journal of Clinical Psychology*, **35**, 505–509.

Grunau, R. V. E., Kearner, S. M. and Whitfield, M. F. (1990) Language development at 3 years in preterm children of birth weight below 1000 g. *The British Journal of Disorders of Communication*, **25**, 173–183.

Gualtieri, C., Koriath, U. V., Van Bourgondieu, M. and Saleeby, N. (1983) Language disorders in children referred for psychiatric services. *American Academy of Child Psychiatry*, **22**, 165–171.

Harris, G. (1986) Barriers to the delivery of speech, language and hearing services to North Americans, in *Nature of Communication Disorders in Culturally and Linguistically Diverse Groups*, (ed. O. Taylor), College Hill Press, San Diego.

Horowitz, F. D. (1982) The first two years of life: factors related to thriving, in *The Young Child Reviews of Research (Vol. 3)*, (eds S. G. Moore and C. R. Cooper), National Association for the Education of Young Children, Washington D. Cox.

Hurst, J. A., Baraitser, M., Auger, E. *et al.* (1990) An extended family with a dominantly inherited speech disorder. *Developmental Medicine and Child Neurology*, **32**, 347–355.

Largo, R. H., Molinari, L., Cemenale Pinto, L. *et al.* (1986) Language development of term and preterm children during the first five years of life. *Developmental Medicine and Child Neurology*, **28**, 333–350.

Lassman, F. M., Fisch, R. O., Vetter, D. K. and La Benz, E. S. (1980) *Early Correlates of Speech, Language and Hearing*, P.S.G. Publishing Company, Littleton, Mass.

Law, J. and Conway, J. (1991) *Child Abuse and Neglect: The Effect on Communication Development – a Review of the Literature*, available from The Association of All Speech Impaired Children, 347 Central Markets, Smithfield, London EC1A 9NH.

Law, J. and Wallfish, T. (1991) Do 'minority' groups have special needs? Speech therapy and the Chasidic Jewish community in north London. *Child: Care, Health and Development*, **17**, 319–329.

Love, A. J. and Thompson, G. G. (1988) Language disorders and attention deficit disorders in young children referred from psychiatric services: Analysis of prevalance and a conceptual synthesis. *American Journal of Orthopsychiatry*, **58** (1), 52–63.

Maccoby, E. and Jacklin, C. (1975) *The Psychology of Sex Differences*, Cambridge University Press, Cambridge.

Mathieson, B., Skuse, D., Wolke, D. and Reily, S. (1989) Oral-motor dysfunction and failure to thrive among inner-city infants. *Developmental Medicine and Child Neurology*, **31**, 293–302.

Mayfield, S. (1983) Language and speech behaviours in children with undue lead absorption: A review of the literature. *Journal of Speech and Hearing Research*, **26**, 362–368.

Mogford, K. and Bishop, D. (1988) Five questions about language acquisition considered in the light of exceptional circumstances, in *Language Development in Exceptional Circumstances*, (eds D. V. M. Bishop and K. Mogford), Churchill Livingstone, Edinburgh, pp. 239–60.

Morley, M. (1972) *The Development and Disorders of Speech in Childhood*, Churchill Livingstone, Edinburgh.

Odebiyi, A. T. (1985) Child rearing practices among nursing mothers in Ife-Ife. Nigeria. *Child: Care Health and Development*, **11**, 325–335.

Puckering, C. and Rutter, M. (1987) Environmental influences on language development, in *Language Development and Disorders*, (eds W. Yule and M. Rutter), MacKeith Press, Oxford, pp. 103–138.

Richman, N., Stevenson, J. and Graham, P. (1982) *Preschool to School: A Behavioural Study*, Academic Press, London.

Robinson, R. (1987) The causes of language disorder – Introduction and overview, in *Proceedings of the First Symposium of Specific Speech and Language Disorders in Children*, Association for All Speech Impaired Children, Middlesex, pp. 1–19.

Rocissano, L. and Yatchmink, Y. (1983) Language skill and interactive patterns in prematurely born toddlers. *Child Development*; **54**, 1229–1241.

Rutter, M. and Madge, N. (1976) *Cycles of Disadvantage*, Heinemann, London.

Schachter, F. F., Shore, E., Hodapp, R. *et al.* (1978) Do girls talk earlier? Mean length of utterance in toddlers. *Developmental Psychology*, **78**, 388–392.

Schery, T. (1985) Correlates of language development in language disordered children. *Journal of Speech and Hearing Disorders*, **50**, 73–83.

Shaywitz, S., Caparilo, B. K. and Hodgson, E. S. (1981) Developmental language disability as a consequence of prenatal exposure to ethanol. *Pediatrics*, **68**, 850–855.

Siegel, L. S. (1982) Reproductive, perinatal and environmental factors as predictors of cognitive and language development of preterm and full term infants. *Child Development*, **53** (4), 963–973.

Silva, P. (1980) The prevalence stability and signifiance of developmental language delay in preschool children. *Developmental Medicine and Child Neurology*, **22**, 768–777.

Silva, P. and Ferguson, D. (1980) Some factors contributing to language development in three-year-old children: A report from the Dunedin Multidisciplinary Child Development Study. *British Journal of Disorders of Communication*, **15**, 205–214.

Skuse, D. (1988) Extreme deprivation in early childhood, in *Language Development in Exceptional Circumstances*. (eds D. Bishop and K. Mogford), Churchill Livingstone, Edinburgh, pp. 29–46.

Snow, C. (1986) Conversations with children, in *Language Acquisition*, (eds P. Fletcher and M. Garman), C.U.P., London, pp. 69–89.

Sparks, S. (1984) *Birth Defects and Speech-Language Disorders*, College Hill Press, San Diego.

Stewart, J., Hester, E. and Taylor, O. (1986) Prevalence of language, speech and hearing disorders in an urban preschool black population *Communication Disorders*, **9** (2), 107–123.

Tallal, P., Ross, R. and Curtiss, S. (1989) Familial aggregation in specific language impairment. *Journal of Speech and Hearing Disorders*, **54**, 167–173.

Yule, W. and Rutter, M. (1987) *Language Development and Disorders*, MacKeith Press, Oxford.

Wanner, E. and Gleitman, L. R. (1986) *Language Acquisition: The State of the Art*, Cambridge University Press, Cambridge.

Widerstrom, A. H., Miller, L. J. and Marzano, R. J. (1986) Sex and race differences in the identification of communication disorders in preschool children as measured by the Miller Assessment for Pre-schoolers. *Journal of Communication Disorders*, **19**, 219–226.

Wulbert, M., Inglis, S. Kriegsman, C. and Mills, B. (1975) Language delay and associated mother/child interactions. *Developmental Psychology*, **11**, 61–70.

4

Behavioural difficulties and their relationship to language impairment

Michael Crowley

The concept of language impairment was introduced in Chapter 2 and the factors commonly associated with it discussed in Chapter 3. In the latter it was observed that one of the most marked associated factors was the high number of language impaired children who presented with behaviour problems – in the region of 50%. This aspect of language impairment is discussed at greater length in the present chapter. In particular it focuses on different possible explanations for the relationship between language and behaviour. The role of parents is emphasized and two theoretical perspectives are offered. The chapter ends with some implications for practice.

THE ASSOCIATION OF DIFFICULTIES IN LANGUAGE AND BEHAVIOUR

In evolutionary terms, the development of speech and of human beings are inextricably interwoven. In the Judeo–Christian myth of Creation the act of 'man' naming creatures is the final integral stage that completes the account. Speech is the attribute which assures humans their place at the head of evolution. In individual terms, human beings develop through their relationships. Once they progress beyond their earliest primitive, dependent relationships and become sophisticated participators in the outside world, children acquire language at an astonishing rate. Yet as we have seen in the last two chapters not only do many children experience difficulties in acquiring language but these same children also have difficulty adjusting to their surroundings. They often present as 'behaviour problems' as preschool children and go on to under-achieve in school.

While it is necessary to identify the processes that might explain the persistent finding that children with language difficulties are at greater risk of developing social and behavioural problems, it is important to recognize that there is no inevitability in this process. Many children, faced with these difficulties, manage to cope admirably well and it would be as instructive to understand how this can happen as to understand why it does not (Griffiths, 1969).

Rutter and Lord (1987) offer the following classification of the possible relationship between language and behaviour.

1. Language difficulties lead to social and emotional problems.
2. Behaviour and emotional problems lead to language difficulties.
3. Both emotional and language difficulties are aspects of the same underlying problem.
4. A common factor causes problems in different ways in both areas.
5. Different factors are causing both sets of problems simultaneously.

Each of these will be considered in turn.

Language difficulties lead to social and emotional problems

In many ways this seems to be the most obvious association. Children who cannot communicate verbally experience frustration and consequently learn to express themselves in other ways. Indeed this does often seem to be the case although there may be some variation according to the type of language difficulty experienced. Thus children with primarily expressive difficulties are less prone to behaviour problems than those with problems of comprehension (Cantwell and Baker, 1987).

It is important, as has already been observed in Chapter 1, that the quality of interaction can make a significant difference to the relationship from the earliest interactions between mother and child. Babies who are unresponsive, who fail to make their presence felt or who never want to communicate, can prove very frustrating for the parents while those who cry persistently or never cease to want to communicate are much more demanding. As the child reaches the age at which peers are beginning to speak, the issue is heightened. If the child is able to recognize needs but is unable to communicate them verbally this means that the parent has to continually take the initiative of interpreting what the child wants. Children with poor communication are less likely to initiate play with their peers, developing a more reactive stance (Siegel *et al.*, 1985). As the child grows older the language delay can affect adversely his relationship with his peers and this, in turn, can result in antisocial behaviour in school.

It is worth noting that the 'behaviour problem' does not necessarily manifest in the type of aggressive externalizing behaviours normally associated with naughty children. It may be that the type of speech/language difficulty determines the behaviour profile (Cantwell and Baker, 1987). Or it may be that extrovert children with limited language skills will tend to act aggressively (see example of Jason below), while more introverted children will tend to become shy and withdrawn.

Case study 4.1

Jason was referred to the child guidance service by his mother when four years old. He had almost no expressive language although he was said to understand well what was said to him. He was demanding and difficult to manage, liable to be angry and aggressive. He attended nursery but the nursery staff frequently commented on his behaviour and his poor language abilities. On occasion they would ask his mother to take him out of the nursery because of his aggression towards other children. His mother was at a loss to know why his speech was so poor and his behaviour so difficult. This was her first child and she could not contemplate having another. Her own mother had had ten children and found it difficult to support her daughter because she couldn't understand how anyone had a difficulty caring for children. Her husband and his family dismissed her concerns, considering Jason no more than high spirited.

Jason continued to attend nursery and simultaneously received help for his expression from the speech therapist. Intervention focused on expanding his expressive vocabulary and encouraging him to express himself using a wider range of grammatical structures. For various reasons no help was forthcoming for his behaviour. Over a period of a year he improved with regular intervention and by 5 years 6 months presented with only minor language difficulties. He continued to be a demanding child but the fact that he could communicate more effectively eased the tension experienced by his mother. He began to form relationships in school and from then on coped reasonably well within the school environment.

Comment: Jason's case is a good example of a child whose difficulty in communicating leads to feelings of powerlessness and a resultant poor behaviour pattern. In his case the latter improved considerably once the former resolved.

Behaviour and emotional problems lead to language difficulties

Bishop (1987), in explaining the causes of developmental language disorder, has suggested that it is highly unlikely that emotional problems cause serious language difficulties. Yet the fact remains that there are a few children who seem to actively resist the use of spoken language. 'Elective mutism' is a clear instance of a condition with its origins in the child's emotional development (Kolvin and Fundudis, 1981). This condition often presents as a persistent, severe and pathological shyness usually manifesting outside the home. It is comparatively rare, with a prevalence of less than one per thousand although this may rise to seven in a thousand when a broader definition is adopted such as 'does not speak to anyone at school at five years' (Brown and Lloyd, 1975). This can be a severe disability and can prove very resistant to intervention. Yet in its milder forms the vast majority of children improve spontaneously. In the Brown and Lloyd study (1975), 90% of children who did not speak at their time of school entry had overcome this by the end of their first year in school.

Within the chronic category, children are invariably excessively shy from an early stage with a great determination not to communicate verbally. They have a tendency to be negative, stubborn and sulky. They are also likely to have some abnormal behaviour, the most common being problems with bowel and bladder control. There is a strong association with low non-verbal intelligence and psychiatric disturbance in other members of the family. Girls are slightly more prone than boys, a factor which is atypical of language difficulties.

Stevenson (1990), too, notes that it is likely that an emotional difficulty is probably only rarely a primary cause of a language impairment. He maintains that it is very likely that the interference of emotional factors exacerbates an existing difficulty with speech and language. In other words it may be wrong to think of the relationship to be a simple one of cause and effect. Rather it may be more useful to see the relationship in terms of a series of interactions between the child and his environment across time.

Both emotional and language difficulties are aspects of the same underlying problem

One example of this type of relationship would be autism in the absence of general developmental delay. Frith (1989) quotes a figure of 25% of all children with autism as having intelligence within the normal range. The aetiology remains elusive. Yet these children manifest both emotional and communication difficulties which are associated with their autistic condition. Furthermore there may be a large group of children who could be said to manifest with 'autistic features'.

These children present as having very little awareness of the meaning of any interaction, show little appreciation of the feelings or intentions of others, do not grasp the importance of the social context of communication, are unable to use language for social communication and, at best, learn only to respond with particular behaviours to associated cues. Lacking any interpretation of their experience which may give some meaning, they over-rely on external order to give their life some coherence. This may reach the point where they become very distraught at minor alterations to details in their lives and they compulsively repeat the same ritual. Similarly they may become extremely attached to certain objects which do not appear to be seen for what they are, but as indispensable extensions of themselves.

Case study 4.2

Gerry was two when he was first referred to speech therapy because his mother had protested to her health visitor that he refused to communicate. Close observation in collaboration with other professionals indicated autism in the absence of other developmental problems. He had, for example, an age-appropriate ability to complete form boards and was able to orientate familiar shapes and patterns without any difficulty. For over a year he continued to receive intervention from a speech therapist and a psychologist together. He responded well to physical games but had no awareness of the meaning of sound. Indeed his lack of response to sound had originally led to a diagnosis of sensori neural hearing loss. Gradually this awareness of sound increased and he would hold his hand to his ear lying on the floor blowing raspberries into his elbow as if feeling his own capacity to perceive sound. For the most part he resisted all eye contact.

From his mother's perspective the problem was primarily social. Although she wanted to know why he was not speaking, her distress reflected their inability to interact effectively. She would infer meaning from his contact but would readily recognize the random quality of much of his interaction. Through the intervention programme she found different ways of relating to him and began to tune into his own agenda. This resulted in them setting up some predictable patterns of interaction – for example a mechanical toy which she would be required to turn on or physical singing games which she taught him to initiate with eye contact. He had still not effectively learned to speak at nine years of age although he was able to imitate some words. His social skills and his understanding of the role of the 'other person' in any interaction did improve, although he continued to have profound problems in this area.

Comment: Gerry's behaviour and language were both manifestations of his autistic condition. Both were highly resistant to change because of the pervasive nature of that condition.

A common factor causes problems in different ways

Children with severe learning difficulties provide an example of this category. Low IQ is the most common cause of psychiatric disturbance, learning difficulties and language delay (Cantwell and Baker, 1987). Their language generally follows a normal course albeit at a retarded rate, but articulation is often poor and they may remain with a limited use of language throughout their lives. Case history 4.3 provides us with an illustration.

Case study 4.3

Barry was fifteen years old and had severe learning difficulties. He was currently attending his third school for children with special needs. Previous schools had not succeeded because his mother felt they were unsympathetic, because Barry himself had a record of being aggressive towards other pupils and because the school felt Barry was not appropriately placed with them.

Barry's speech remained very limited and had not developed at all over the past few years. He was overweight because his mother felt food was one of his few pleasures in life and she found it hard to refuse his demands. Barry hit and kicked his mother and frequently resorted to damaging the flat.

Barry's disability was apparent at birth. From that point Barry's father had taken no interest in his son. His mother's family found her demands too great and only her own mother helped out. Barry's mother felt that her son's disability was the price she had to pay for his illegitimacy. Even though, at times, she wished to escape from him she also felt she must lie on the bed she has made and after many years of Barry's total dependency she now had few interests outside her home.

Barry and his mother have received a considerable amount of help in the form of extra activities for Barry outside school, respite care for Barry and individual help for his mother who has also joined a self-help group. Although the difficulties have eased as Barry has gained personal independence, they will need further help for some time. In Barry's case his overwhelming developmental difficulties underlie all his skills.

Comment: It is impossible to disentangle the effects of Barry's communication difficulties, his frustrated behaviours and his overall development.

Different factors cause different problems simultaneously

There may be any number of different factors, social deprivation, shyness, developmental problems, etc. which may together interact to produce both psychological and emotional problems. This corresponds to the multivariate model outlined in Chapter 2 and probably best approximates the situation in most clinical conditions.

Case study 4.4

Jane had been attending a language unit for a year and was now five. When she started in the unit she had almost no speech and required constant attention and supervision. Some of the staff in the unit considered her difficulties to be primarily language related while others felt her emotional disturbance were the basis of her problems. She formed a very close relationship with her teacher who challenged the view that Jane was primarily a disturbed child. The situation was complicated by a history of ear infections although the audiology clinic maintained that there were no outstanding difficulties in this area. Her mother considered her 'a great handful' but felt that the school should be able to manage her.

The family lived on benefit which left them with little practical resources. Jane's parents had a violent relationship. More recently this had calmed down because they saw less of each other. Jane's mother was very overweight. Her children were important to her but there was constant friction between them. Jane had an older brother and sister. The latter was also critically overweight, messed herself and smeared her faeces in the home.

Comment: It is impossible to put Jane's difficulties down to neurodevelopmental, medical or environmental causes. Her experience is the product of a complex interaction of the three. Although she may be integrated back into mainstream school it is likely that she will continue to have schooling difficulties.

THE ROLE OF THE PARENTS

As already observed in Chapter 3, parents are intricately linked into the experience of language impairment both because of the family nature of many of the difficulties and because it is to them that professionals turn in the process of their assessments and their intervention.

Just as the experience of having a child with a physical handicap will dramatically affect that child's family, it is also important to try and understand the family's possible reaction to a child with communication difficulties. The realization that their child has a disability (which may be permanent and profound) involves the sadness of grieving for the child that might have been. The pain of grief (disbelief, overwhelming sadness, looking for an explanation, self-blame) is, hopefully, followed by a period of adjustment. However difficult this may be, this is a human response to loss. Parents have to live through this while continuing to cope with their handicapped child. It is important to recognize that other children in the family are also involved in this proces of adjustment.

In the case of the language impaired child, the child may look normal but be relatively unresponsive. Some mothers report that their care for their baby became mechanical and unrewarding in such circumstances. It is common for families in this position to experience considerable stress and difficulty. Possibly the fact that the difficulties are not as obvious as those associated with other handicaps makes the situation worse for the families concerned.

In some instances parents and carers may abandon all attempts to control the child's behaviour by speech and thereby further negate the child's capacity to communicate. In such situations no attempt is made to explain why a behaviour is inappropriate or wrong. Conversely, some children acquire an apparent sophistication in one aspect of their lives and this may result in the adult having too high an expectation of the child's overall skills, leading to an inappropriate level of language being directed to the child. Talking over the child's head in this way can be just as undermining for the child as a parent's reluctance to use language at all.

In the final analysis the parent is likely to be by far and away the most important person in any child's life. For this reason any intervention will necessarily focus on the parent as the vehicle for treatment. This may prove complex especially if the parent is felt to be contributing to the child's difficulties. Yet without the involvement of the parent little can be achieved.

THE PSYCHODYNAMIC PERSPECTIVE

The next two sections highlight two very different approaches to accounting for the relationship between behaviour, emotional development and language. As we have seen at the beginning of Chapter 1, the increased sophistication in research methods has added to our knowledge of very early cognitive development by emphasizing the skills which the infant possesses early in life. Developments in psychoanalytic thinking have also emphasized the power of tiny infants to influence their surroundings emotionally. Both these approaches emphasize the view that neither the emotional nor the cognitive life of a child is merely a reaction to life experiences. Even the very small infant is seen as having considerable psychological resources and skills with which to interact with their environment.

However, beyond this emphasis on the role of the very young child, theories of children's emotional and cognitive development have remained very separate, mirroring splits between reason and emotion, body and mind, so pervasive in Western culture. There has therefore been little interchange between these separate theories beyond a recognition that the one aspect is part of the context within which the other develops. It is important to consider a psychoanalytic perspective[1] partly because it presents a well-developed view of the emotional life of children at the time they are acquiring preverbal and verbal skills. It offers an understanding of a dynamic relationship between the development of the capacity to use symbols and the emotional growth of the individual.

Within the psychoanalytic view, the baby appreciates its vulnerable state within the first few months of life and experiences corresponding feelings of overwhelming anxiety. Psychological survival is only achieved through the use of 'defence mechanisms' which, at this stage, involve distorting the perception of reality to render it less threatening. Thus some aspects of reality are denied, conflicting feelings are kept apart, unwelcome feelings are displaced onto others and some aspects from outside are appropriated as belonging to oneself. While this distorts and confuses reality it does create a world in which it is possible to live. In some ways the infant can be seen to be re-ordering his world in a rather magical way by creating a fantasy world (which he or she takes to be real).

This phase gives way to a stage (at about four to five months) in which reality begins to be accepted to a greater extent. This is facilitated by the reassurance of reliable carers and is also made possible by increasing cognitive skills which make his world a less threatening place. The person who is giving is also recognized as the person who withholds. Instead of conflicting feelings being kept rigorously apart, some integration is allowed and ambivalent feelings are tolerated. Thus the infant simultaneously finds himself wishing to attack the same thing that he loves (i.e. the parent). The previous stage was characterized by feelings of persecution, with the infant attacking an object which he perceived as totally threatening and real (even though it was of his own creation). With some awareness that the object that he attacks is also the object he loves, his predominant feeling is guilt. The only way of coping with this guilt is to make good by reparation.

For the resolution of these feelings of destruction and the ensuing restoration of the parent, the infant needs to differentiate between his psychic reality and external reality. He needs to appreciate that the world he creates and destroys is not the outside world but his world of fantasy, and that they have a separate,

---

[1] There is an extensive literature dealing with psychodynamic theory. Here I refer to what has become known as the 'object relations' school normally associated with the writings of Melanie Klein. The reader is referred to Segal (1986a and 1986b) for further discussion.

though related existence. He needs to maintain his inner world as a means of coping and for this he needs symbols to represent his perception of reality. This is the development of consciousness, of self-awareness in which symbols, while being related to the external world, also have an independent existence of their own in the internal world of the child. With the development of symbols comes the ability to be aware of oneself, to communicate with oneself, and this is the basis of verbal thinking.

It is this ability to construct a world of symbols that is 'real', while recognizing that it is not the reality of the external world, that enables us to develop fiction, the theatre, and other belief systems. One of the earliest forms of symbolic representation is the 'comfort' (e.g. a teddy bear) of a small child. Both the parent and the child accept at some level that the object, in itself, is of little value. However, it is invested with special significance so that the symbol alone may be sufficient to comfort the child (Winnicott, 1971).

This second phase follows once the child comes to accept reality for what it is. It is possible to see that this process continues throughout our lives. Mature people have learnt to live with themselves as they are. This process extends beyond our perception to our view of the world. Some would argue that religion is nothing more than a world of symbols, a construction of our psyche, while others would maintain it exists in reality outside our minds. Within this framework, the person who cannot distinguish between symbol and reality can be described as 'psychotic'. An autistic child can be seen as one who does not have an inner and outer world. There is therefore no communication and no construction of meaning. Without the use of symbols there is no possibility for the development of language.

In summary, the psychodynamic perspective offers us one possible explanation for the relationship between the breakdown in the attachment process in the first year of life and subsequent language problems. Thus the child's difficulty in learning to symbolize the parent becomes translated into difficulties in other aspects of symbolic ability. As we have seen in Chapter 2, it is this symbolic capacity which appears to underlie subsequent difficulties in both play and language development. This perspective also helps us to explain how difficult it is without language to separate from the parent, to allow the self to develop fully.

THE ECOLOGICAL PERSPECTIVE

If the psychodynamic perspective focuses on the processes internal to the child the ecological perspective emphasizes the child's external reality. Indeed the ecological view rests on the assumption that within any system all the component parts are mutually interdependent. Originally developed as a theoretical perspective for simple biological systems, it was quickly seen to have relevance for human groups (Campion, 1985). People can be regarded as systems with their own sub-systems (such as various biological and psychological systems) and are themselves part of larger systems (such as families, societies, religions). How these systems interact can be observed and at a more abstract level it is possible to identify properties common to all systems and rules common to all interactions between systems.

There are two essential components to the theory. The first is that causality is seen as circular rather than linear. It is not that there is a primary cause which creates change, rather like the billiard ball which hits all the others and creates a new relationship between all the balls. Rather the relationship between the component parts is in a constant state of flux. The other characteristic of particular interest here is that systems are seen as continually acting to preserve and maintain themselves in a state of equilibrium by adjusting their internal and external relationships. For example a trade union can be seen as a system and all its activities of seeking allies, expelling some members, recruiting others, seeking conflict with one system and avoiding it with another, can all be understood in this light.

When applied to a clinical setting the task is to understand how a series of systems are interacting together for a given child. To do so it is necessary to understand how the individual's biological, cognitive and psychological systems interact with other systems such as the family, the educational and the medical systems which in turn interact with the system of the therapist. The purpose is to redress whatever imbalance is apparent. One solution is to expand the system or include another system. In other words, the therapist or teacher assumes that in any referral there is a state of disequilibrium between or within systems that the inclusion of the third system (the therapist's) is intended to resolve.

The therapist, the health visitor or the teacher are likely to have become involved at this level because the existing systems have failed to establish equilibrium. However, many adaptations

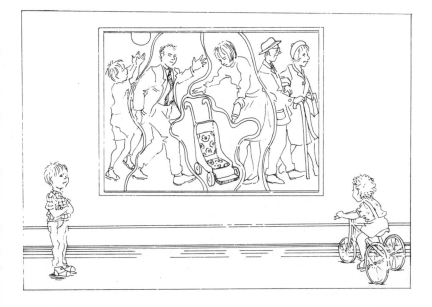

and adjustments will already have occurred to ensure some compromise between conflicting systems in order to achieve this equilibrium. Children may have learned other ways of communicating that do not involve language and other members of the family may, in turn, have learned how to interpret their communication. Families may find idiosyncratic ways of coping with their disabled child. Sometimes there may be massive upheaval with siblings taking on considerable responsibilities, parents leaving their jobs or moving home to be near better resources.

Families and individuals are better equipped to deal with a 'different' child where they are flexible in finding a suitable response. Individuals and families that are over-determined and have a limited range of responses to a new situation are less able to adapt and cope. For example, a parent who is very capable and coping is a tremendous asset in a family under stress. But if

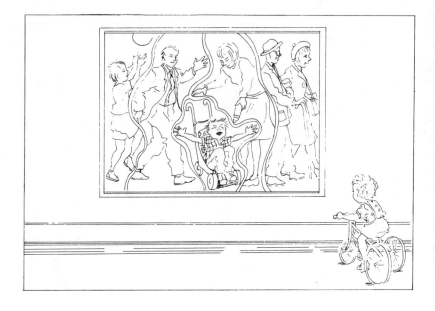

he or she is never anything but capable and coping in times of stress this can be a liability, because everyone around them will be made to feel correspondingly useless. Furthermore there may be no way of knowing if this person is close to breaking point.

From this perspective it is best to view difference and abnormality in families where there is a person with a language difficulty as an ability to respond to change in circumstances. For example, where there is a child with a severe disability one parent may give up work and become extremely involved in the care of that child. Yet this may be to the detriment of other aspects of their own life, for example in excluding their other children who, in turn, will feel left out. This may be a functional solution to threatened disequilibrium and other aspects of the system may adapt successfully to accommodate (for example other members of the family may support this parent in their role and seek more interests for themselves outside the family). If we consider this an 'unhealthy' response it may be that we are less flexible in responding to an unusual predicament than the family we see. We may also be more unwilling than they to recognize the reality of the extent to which a disabled person disrupts 'normal' life.

However, where adaptations to a young person in difficulty are seen to be unhelpful, it is necessary to determine whether these adaptations do serve a function. For example, although two parents may never agree on the extent to which they should make demands on their language impaired child and constantly argue over the management of the child, this may serve the function of distracting from other conflicts which would pose a greater threat to their relationship. Faced with the dilemma of whether to leave their child caught between parental conflict or expose themselves to the possibility of irresolvable marital tension, the system has opted for the solution that provides greater equilibrium.

There may be aspects of the way that systems have adapted to each other that are considered inadequate, but which have fulfilled the function of reducing disequilibrium. If the therapist's system seeks to change this, the system will be threatened by disequilibrium and will resist intervention. For example, a child with communication difficulties may be placed with an elderly grandmother partly because the grandmother is lonely and a burden to her family. Much as the parents want the therapist to help with their child's difficulties, they will resist suggestions that their child is placed in a more stimulating environment.

The involvement of the therapist's system may itself reduce the disequilibrium. For example, if there is a conflict between a school and parents over whether a young person has a language difficulty or a behaviour problem, by producing a formulation that satisfies both sides, equilibrium is restored. There may be only a polite interest in any recommended intervention which somehow never gets implemented. By producing a formulation similar to that of the school, the therapist has failed to resolve the conflict and the parents will have to find another system to fulfil this function. It is always as well to have an open mind about the function of intervention and how this may conflict with a professional role. Examples of this are probably very familiar. The therapist may be required to continue to treat a child because another system needs to continue to see the child as 'having problems', or where the function of treatment may be to provide surrogate parenting.

From a more positive viewpoint, this approach emphasizes how any change in one part of the system will affect changes throughout the system. For example, improving the relationship between the child and the teacher will improve the child's chances of learning, the parents are likely to have a more positive attitude towards both the child and the school, the child's self-esteem will improve, the teacher will be encouraged by progress in the child and by the parents' increased support and so on.

IMPLICATIONS FOR PRACTICE

In Chapter 2 we saw how difficult it was to be clinically sure as to our definition of language impairment. The same is also true of 'behaviour problem'. Although it is possible to use checklists which have been standardized, in practice their application is usually confined to research projects. Instead professionals make judgements as to what does or does not constitute a problem according to their own preconceptions and experience coupled with a measure of the relative anxiety of parents and other professionals. The following are some areas which need to be considered in any intervention offered to language impaired children both with and without behaviour problems. They should be taken in conjunction with the comments made in Chapter 8 specifically relating to intervention for language impaired children.

Resources

Clearly from the discussion in Chapters 2 and 3 there are a great many factors to be considered when offering treatment to these children. Because these factors are so closely interrelated it is often necessary to provide a range of integrated services. Where such services are not co-ordinated there is a need to improve organizational relationships and working practices. From the client's point of view, it may be that the fewer the professionals that are involved the better. For example, a psychotherapist might consider it a more economical use of time to advise a speech therapist already involved on some emotional aspects of a child's life. The client would benefit both by only having to see one professional and also by not having to acquire a label of 'emotional difficulties' in order to be referred to the psychotherapist.

Integration of services necessarily raises the issue of how far one profession should 'transgress' its own area of expertise and involve itself in areas that properly belong to other professions. This problem is usually more related to the quality of existing inter-professional relationships than theoretical issues. Where these are good, professions discuss clients together at an early stage, make joint decisions on how to integrate their work and respect each other's differences and expertise.

Assessment phase

Given the interaction between behaviour and language it is hardly surprising that children with equivalent problems may be referred to child guidance or to speech therapy services. In both cases care should be taken to ensure that assessment includes both aspects of the child's development. Thus the speech therapist needs to consider the personal and social implications for the child while the child guidance worker needs to assess the child's language ability. It is not enough to assume that by helping with a primary language difficulty other problems will not arise or will spontaneously disappear. Similarly psychotherapy or counselling makes no sense without an understanding of the child's linguistic abilities.

Although different types of difficulties frequently present together, it is necessary to carefully examine their relationship. It is possible to mistake the reaction to a difficulty with its cause. For example, a parent's limited use of vocabulary may be a response to their child's limited ability to understand rather than the cause of their child's limited understanding of their world. It is unwise to presume that abnormalities in the child's environment are necessarily unhelpful. Rather it may be more useful to assume that they are the best solution that could be found at the time and your understanding will need to take account of the function this abnormality serves.

Intervention

Some children with language difficulties have profound psychological difficulties or severe learning difficulties which will remain largely unaltered by the best care and treatment. They may make tremendous demands on their carers throughout their lives. It is probably best to act in as straightforward a manner as possible in informing parents of their child's strengths and weaknesses. Knowing is better than being uncertain about what they have to deal with and parents should be given information at the earliest opportunity. Equally it is best to be straight about not knowing answers (even when you think you should) and to ensure all information is given in a way that can be understood by these particular parents respecting their culture, beliefs, their intelligence and knowledge. It is imperative that a collaborative relationship between parents and professionals is established and maintained and much work may have to be invested in this.

Dealing with parental denial of difficulties where serious problems have been identified can be extremely difficult, not least because it can leave the worker feeling exasperated and angry to the point where professional judgement is threatened by personal issues. Perhaps it is as well to remember that denial is a very primitive defence, used as a last resort when people feel profoundly threatened. Almost certainly, the more evidence for 'problems' is presented, the more entrenched will become their position. Positions will become equally hardened on both sides, with neither able to assimilate new evidence. Being able to identify their child's difficulty may lead the family to invest the professional with many other qualities which they hope will enable them to improve matters. Over-confidence in professional expertise can be used therapeutically. It should, at least, reduce anxiety and this is usually helpful. It may also mean clients will more readily comply with treatment plans. Yet there may be a corresponding undervaluing of their own potential in contributing to improving matters. In all these matters self-help groups can help enormously by validating the experience of clients, counteracting feelings of dependency and powerlessness, offering practical support and advice, providing an opportunity for feeling profoundly understood and an environment in which the children are not made to feel different. They are frequently able to provide immediate help and relief in times of crisis.

Whether they like it or not, all professionals are involved in the social and emotional aspects of their clients' lives. The skilled professional will be aware of some of the implications of these aspects and seek to change attitudes, behaviours and relations as they consider in their clients' interests. Part of our professional responsibility is to understand how our personal feelings and biases might affect our professional decisions and dealings with people. Moreover, part of our skill lies in our ability to create an environment within which people can share their concerns, can learn and develop. We have to create an emotional environment within which this is possible and for this we rely on the professional development of our personal skills. Of course, we also have some personal investment in succeeding in our work. We hope it will provide some satisfaction. While our clients rely on us to be professional and put their requirements first, they also require us to contribute personally to our work. While some professionals may relish the opportunity to become more involved in their clients' emotional and social lives, others may feel it inappropriate (for themselves or for their colleagues) to be involved in this way.

SUMMARY AND CONCLUSIONS

In summary the following points can be taken from the text of this chapter.

- In cultural terms it is almost inevitable that language and behaviour will be inextricably linked. A substantial proportion of children experiencing problems in one area will also experience difficulties in another.
- The most common explanation of the direction of the relationship between behaviour and language is that problems in the latter lead to difficulties with the former. There are a number of other possible explanations which need to be borne in mind.
- Of particular interest are the reasons that some children do not present with behavioural difficulties in spite of their linguistic difficulties.
- Parental perception of the child's difficulties together with an evaluation of the parent's capacity to respond to intervention is an integral part of the understanding of the relationship between behaviour and language difficulties.
- The psychodynamic perspective offers insight into the internal world of the child. In this model there is a predictable link between the child's inability to symbolically represent the mother and subsequent difficulties in manipulating conventional symbolic systems of which language is the prime example.
- Equally the ecological perspective allows us to examine the relationship both of the child to the family and of the child

to any system of intervention. Care must be taken to determine in whose interest it is to effect change.

● Intervention relies on all those involved understanding the relationship between behaviour and language development in the individual case.

If the implication of this chapter is that professionals working with people with language difficulties take a closer look at the emotional and social lives of their clients, there is a corresponding implication that professionals consider their own personal attitudes and the emotional commitment that they bring to their work. From the point of view of the early identification of language impaired children it is imperative that the process includes an assessment of emotional development and behaviour. It is likely that the child who exhibits both a delay in the acquisition of language skills and poor behaviour is particularly vulnerable in terms of his future development.

REFERENCES

Bishop, D. V. M. (1987) The causes of developmental language disorder (developmental dysphasia). *Journal of Psychology and Psychiatry*, **28** (1), 1–8.

Brown, J. B. and Lloyd, H. (1975) A controlled study of children not speaking at school. *Journal of Association of Workers with Maladjusted Children*, **3**.

Campion, J. (1985) *The Child in Context*, Methuen, London.

Cantwell, D. P. and Baker, L. (1987) Prevalence and type of psychiatric disorders in three speech and language groups. *Journal of Communication Disorders*, **20**, 151–160.

Frith, U. (1989) *Autism: Explaining the Enigma*, Blackwell, Oxford.

Griffiths, C. (1969) A follow up study of children with disorders of speech. *British Journal of Disorders of Communication*, **4**, 46–56.

Kolvin, I. and Fundudis, T. (1981) Elective mute children: Psychological development and background factors. *Journal of Child Psychology and Psychiatry*, **22** (3), 219–232.

Rutter, M. and Lord, C. (1987) Language disorders associated wiith psychiatric disturbance, in *Language Development and Disorders*, (eds W. Yule and M. Rutter) MacKeith Press, Oxford, pp. 206–233.

Siegel, L. S., Cunningham, C. E. and van der Spuy, H. I. J. (1985) Interactions of language delayed and normal preschool boys with their peers. *Journal of Child Psychology and Psychiatry*, **26**, 77–83.

Segal, H. (1986a) *Delusion and Artistic Creativity and Other Psychoanalytic Essays*, Free Association Books, London.

Segal, H. (1986b) *Introduction to the Work of Melanie Klein*, Hogarth, London.

Stevenson, J. (1990) The relationship between emotional/behaviour problems and communication difficulties in young children. Paper presented at the Annual Conference of the Association for Child Psychology and Psychiatry, June 1990.

Winnicott, D. (1971) *Playing and Reality*, Tavistock, London.

5

The early identification of hearing loss and the effects of impaired hearing on language development

Rosemary Emanuel and Ros Herman

In the previous chapter specific attention was drawn to the relationship between language development and behaviour. This chapter sets out to investigate the problems that may arise when hearing is impaired. In order to prevent some of these problems and minimize others, it is important to detect the presence of a hearing loss as early as possible. Families and health care professionals have a significant role to play in the assessment of hearing in young children. When a hearing loss is suspected, referral to a hearing assessment clinic will allow an in-depth investigation to take place, both of the child's hearing status and of the underlying causes of any hearing deficits. Among other things, this involves the use of diagnostic tests which are appropriate to the child's developmental level. We have therefore included a brief outline of the various audiological assessment procedures appropriate to children at different stages in their development. For reference a brief outline of the role of hearing in infant development is given in Chapter 1 and there is a diagram of the structure of the ear in Appendix A.

TYPES OF HEARING LOSS

Hearing losses are usually described according to the site of lesion. Any problem of transmission of sound through the outer or middle ear causes a **conductive hearing loss**. With this type of loss, incoming sound loses intensity, but because all frequencies tend to be fairly evenly affected, sounds are perceived as quieter but relatively undistorted. The effects of a slight conductive loss can be simulated by occluding the ear canals with the finger tips. The degree of loss will vary according to the nature and severity of the pathology. Most conductive losses are remediable, either by medical or surgical treatment.

Where the pathology lies in the inner ear or the auditory nerve, the term **sensori-neural hearing loss** is used. The hearing loss is permanent and although much can be done to reduce its impact, there are no medical or surgical remedies. A sensori-neural hearing loss is usually more severe for high frequency sounds than for those of lower frequency. This imbalance causes distortion and clarity is not necessarily improved by an increase in the intensity of speech. The effects of such distortion can be experienced to some degree when listening to conversation in an adjoining room. Even when voices are raised in intensity such that intonation patterns are clearly perceived, because important high frequency information has been filtered out by the wall, the conversation cannot be understood.

Some people with sensori-neural loss, particularly of cochlear origin, may be unable to perceive quiet sounds, yet may find more intense sounds intolerably loud. This phenomenon, called **recruitment**, may present a problem when amplification is needed.

Of course, a hearing loss may have both conductive and sensori-neural components. In such **mixed losses** it is important to identify the relative contribution of each pathology to ensure appropriate management.

Some children may have apparent difficulties in listening and in deriving meaning from sound, particularly the complexities of spoken language. After careful assessment their hearing acuity is found to be normal. This inability to interpret and integrate auditory information has sometimes been labelled **central deafness**, or **central auditory dysfunction**. In this chapter, however, we are confining our discussion to those children with identifiable peripheral hearing loss.

The hearing mechanism is vulnerable to damage at any stage in our lives, from events prior to conception, to those occurring in old age. Below we consider some of the more common causes of impaired hearing in young children (see Northern and Downs, 1984, for a more detailed discussion of this area).

CAUSES OF CONDUCTIVE AND SENSORI-NEURAL HEARING LOSS IN CHILDREN

Causes of conductive hearing loss

Although a conductive loss is rarely severe, it may in certain circumstances lead to difficulties ranging from poor behaviour to delayed language development. It is also this category of hearing loss which occurs in babies and young children, and so the common causes of conductive deafness deserve special mention.

Infection

Conductive deafness is most often a consequence of an infection in the middle ear, otitis media and 80% of children have had at least one attack before the age of five (McCormick, 1988). Otitis media may arise as a complication of a cold, throat infection, or 'flu virus. Infection from the upper respiratory tract spreads easily to the Eustachian tubes, which are shorter and more horizontal than those of adults. These then provide a channel for infection to extend to the middle ear. The lining of the middle ear becomes swollen and infected and produces pus. The build-up of pressure due to pus may, in severe cases, cause the eardrum to burst. The conductive loss is thus a result of alterations to the mobility of the middle ear mechanism.

Most cases of otitis media resolve, often with the help of antibiotics. In some cases, the condition is chronic, with fluid remaining in the middle ear space. As a result, the hearing loss persists and surgical intervention is necessary to artificially ventilate the middle ear.

Serious otitis media, or glue ear, may be related to attacks of acute otitis media, or may occur in children whose Eustachian tubes function inefficiently. In these circumstances, a viscous sterile fluid is produced by the mucous membrane lining and remains in the middle ear for an extended period of months or even years. The resultant hearing loss often varies widely and this inconsistency manifests itself in behavioural, communication and educational difficulties.

Genetic factors

Conductive deafness is associated with over half of all cases of Down's syndrome (Downs, 1980). External ear abnormalities and unusual nasopharynx and Eustachian tube development contribute to this finding. In addition, middle ear infection has been found to be particularly persistent in this population (Balkany, 1980) even after medical or surgical intervention, and this may in turn lead to chronic ear disease.

Structural abnormalities in the outer or middle ear are known to occur frequently in syndromes characterized by cranio-facial anomalies. The high incidence of hearing problems associated with cleft palate is thought to be due to poor palatal musculature which is insufficient to maintain adequate Eustachian tube function (Bluestone and Shurin, 1974). The ears of all children with these syndromes need to be regularly examined for signs of middle ear disease and subsequent hearing loss, although the incidence and severity of these problems often decrease as the children grow older.

Occlusion of the outer ear

In children this generally refers to the presence of a foreign body (e.g. a bead) or the build-up of wax, both of which are removable, thereby restoring normal hearing.

Causes of sensori-neural hearing loss

Genetic factors

At least half of all cases of sensori-neural deafness are thought to be due to genetic factors. That is not to say that deaf children are generally born into families where deafness is commonplace. Indeed the converse is more often true, with one or both parents being carriers of the responsible gene without being affected themselves. Deafness may also be part of the cluster of symptoms associated with particular syndromes, e.g. Waardenburg's syndrome and Usher's syndrome.

Infection and trauma

During pregnancy, the developing foetus is susceptible to maternal infection by certain viruses, such as rubella. Where rubella is contracted within the first trimester, the risk of the child being affected is high. Among the handicaps which may result is a severe impairment of hearing caused by damage to the inner ear. The rubella epidemic of the 1960s led to an alarming increase in the numbers of deaf and multiply handicapped children being born. Subsequent rubella vaccination programmes and monitoring for rubella infection in the antenatal period have been effective in reducing these numbers, although among groups which have not been vaccinated rubella is still a common cause of sensori-neural deafness.

Difficulties at the time of birth may result in damage to the hearing mechanism. For example, where the baby is starved of oxygen, the delicate hair cells in the inner ear may be affected. Severe jaundice at or around the time of birth may also cause this type of deafness. Sensori-neural deafness may be acquired in later years due to infection (e.g. meningitis), trauma or the use of ototoxic drugs. In general, the later the age of onset and the more moderate the loss, the better the prognosis.

WHAT CONSTITUTES A SIGNIFICANT HEARING LOSS?

We have already observed the difficulties inherent in defining the language impaired population. Similarly, although various degrees of severity of hearing loss have been identified, the precise point at which a hearing loss becomes significant for an individual child has not really been established (Northern and Downs, 1984).

Certainly, the 25 dB threshold which normally defines the beginning of hearing loss in adults is insufficiently stringent to demarcate the minimum critical level for a child's hearing threshold. This is because of the importance of hearing for speech at different ages. An adult who is already familiar with the linguistic system can compensate for distortions to the spoken message. A child, who is in the process of acquiring language, needs to hear particularly acutely in order to extrapolate the speech system from background noise, and from the variability which exists between speakers of the same language. Furthermore, the acoustic make-up of speech sounds renders certain of them vulnerable to distortion from even a 10 dB hearing loss. Even a slight unilateral loss (Bess, 1982) can have handicapping linguistic, educational and behavioural effects on a young child.

Northern and Downs propose the following definition: 'a handicapping hearing loss in a child is any degree of hearing that reduces the intelligibility of a speech message to a degree inadequate for accurate interpretation or learning'. A virtue inherent in such a definition is that it does not attempt to delimit the precise factors which inhibit an individual child's ability to learn. This is difficult to do because of the number of potential variables which may be present and which relate to the individual child and his environment. Northern and Downs suggest that it is up to the professionals involved to determine whether or not a hearing loss is affecting a child's language learning.

WHAT ARE THE POSSIBLE DAMAGING EFFECTS OF A HEARING LOSS?

The majority of conductive hearing losses are neither severe nor irreversible. However, if left untreated, a slight conductive loss can have detrimental effects on the young child acquiring language. Research studies have shown speech discrimination to be impaired in children with a history of otitis media (e.g. Dobie and Berlin, 1979). Even when speech discrimination appears normal in quiet situations, it is likely that performance will be reduced where listening conditions are less than ideal (Jerger *et al.*, 1983). Moreover, these effects are exacerbated by the fluctuating nature of middle ear infections and the interaction of other predisposing factors, where present. Bishop and Edmundson (1986) noted that the consequences of otitis media may be particularly serious 'where a child is particularly vulnerable for developing language disorders, because of genetic predisposition, poor environment, or brain damage'.

Other studies have identified negative effects on language as measured by vocabulary tests and tests of auditory comprehension (e.g. Teele *et al.*, 1981). Such effects have been found to be particularly in evidence where the conductive loss occurred in the first six months of life, and may be more marked among children from lower socio-economic groups. Such effects have been shown to have consequences for later educational achievement (see Northern and Downs, 1984, for a more detailed account).

Sensori-neural deafness ranges from moderate to profound in degree, and is permanent. Depending on the impairment of discrimination ability which results and the presence of other factors, the effects on the process of language acquisition, and on learning which occurs via language, may be very variable. At one extreme, the bright child with only a moderate loss and a supportive home and school environment may do extremely well, with only residual speech and language difficulties. The less advantaged child with an equivalent loss may have considerable language deficits, exhibit behavioural problems, and seriously underachieve at school.

Many children with profound sensori-neural deafness fail to master spoken language at all, although they are able to learn effectively when exposed to alternative forms of communication (sign language). For the purposes of the present text, these children represent a small minority about which there is a separate literature, and so will not be addressed further here.

Where either a conductive or a sensori-neural hearing loss is present, it is not the capacity to learn language, but rather the capacity to access spoken language which is impaired. In cases where the loss fluctuates, access is inconsistent and the effects on auditory skills may be surprisingly damaging. With appropriate early intervention, access may be facilitated during the critical years for language acquisition, thereby minimizing the effects of the hearing loss. It is therefore of prime importance to detect the presence of a hearing loss as early as possible, in order to implement such intervention.

In the next two sections we look at the ways in which a hearing loss can be detected. Later in the chapter we consider how the detrimental effects of impaired hearing may be minimized.

HEARING EVALUATION

For a child's language skills to develop normally and easily, he must be able to hear all the important elements of quiet speech, even in noisy listening situations. To do this, a child needs to be able to hear sounds, bilaterally, of an intensity level of 20 dB or less across the sound frequency range important for speech perception. (A young adult with above-average hearing will have a threshold of acuity of 0 dB; in normal conversation, speech sounds may reach an average intensity of 40–60 dB.)

An effective screening programme should identify all those children whose hearing does not meet this criterion. Although the importance of early identification has long been recognized, the establishment of an effective screening programme poses many problems. Since hearing ability may fluctuate or deteriorate, assessment must be repeated.

Neonatal procedures

Ideally, the first tests of hearing 'adequacy' should be given before newborn babies leave hospital. Opinions differ as to whether all babies should be tested (as advocated by Tucker, 1986), or whether there should be selective screening of babies in special-care units where the highest risk of deafness exists.

Most procedures developed for neonates have attempted to measure behavioural responses to sounds, such as changes in respiration, heartbeat, sucking, body movement. Two such auto-mated procedures which utilize a microprocessor are the 'cribo-gram' (Simmons and Russ, 1974) and the 'auditory response cradle' (Bennett, 1975). The cribogram contains a pressure-sensitive transducer, sensitive to the baby's movement. The auditory response cradle records head turns, body movements and respiratory changes. Both procedures use narrow band noise centred at around 3000 Hertz presented at 85–92 dB SPL.

Although results of studies are variable, there are a number of problems with such procedures. The systems are expensive in that they yield a high rate of false positive responses and are insufficiently sensitive to identify all significant losses. The results are found to be particularly unreliable with 'special care' babies.

Alternatives to behavioural techniques are likely to provide greater reliability and give a more accurate indication of hearing acuity, but only assess the more peripheral hearing function. The measurement of auditory brainstem evoked responses (ABR) involves the recording and computer analysis of EEG signals evoked in response to 'clicks'. This test provides useful information about hearing function as far as the brain stem. Another procedure, developed more recently, records stimulated oto-acoustic emissions (weak echoes from the cochlea), which are present in all ears with normal hearing function, but which are very weak or absent in those with losses in excess of 30 dB (Stevens *et al.*, 1987). Although more trials are needed, both these approaches offer a potentially viable means of screening the hearing even of special-care infants.

Recent developments in neonatal tests are promising, but at present their use is mainly for selective screening of high-risk infants and as a research procedure.

The 6–8 months screening test

Although babies 'at risk' may have their hearing responses carefully monitored throughout their first months, the majority of infants will continue with little consideration of hearing until approximately seven months, when (in the UK) a routine screening test is administered by health visitors. This 'distraction' test requires that the baby make a clear turning response to a range of high, middle and low frequency sounds presented to each side of the child on a horizontal plane at low intensities (not more than 35 dB). Babies who respond adequately to this test are considered to be without serious hearing disability; those who 'fail' on two occasions are referred for further assessment to the audiology clinic.

However, a poor response to this test does not necessarily imply hearing impairment; there are many reasons other than deafness which may cause a child to be referred. Some children referred for re-assessment are subsequently found to respond entirely normally and for a small number of babies, their poor response to sound may be indicative of other developmental difficulties.

Because of the difficulty in standardizing such 'free-field' procedures, their validity, reliability and consequently the value of the distraction test has been questioned. Obviously test efficacy varies considerably. One study showed that only 20% of the babies later diagnosed as congenitally deaf were identified by this test. Subsequently, in that district, the rate of accurate identification of deaf babies was increased dramatically, to over 70%. This improvement was effected by better health visitor training, by careful calibration and standardization of test stimuli and procedure and the routine use of parental questionnaires devised to increase awareness of potential pointers to hearing difficulty (McCormick, 1988). It has been shown (Hitchings and Haggard, 1983) that parental estimations of their children's hearing abilities are usually accurate and should be routinely incorporated into the screening programme.

Screening tests for infants over twelve months old

There are difficulties in the administration of the 'distraction' test to older infants, as they develop more sophisticated listening behaviour and are selective about the sounds which interest them. They are therefore less willing to turn repeatedly and it requires an experienced tester and modified techniques to obtain an accurate result.

For children over eighteen months, additional tests are used; suitable screening procedures for older infants are included below in the section on diagnostic tests. Unless doubt about hearing is expressed, or potential problems noted, specific tests of hearing are not routinely administered (in the UK) between nine months and five years of age.

Intermediate screening specifically for hearing loss is not seen as justifiable at present (Hall, 1989; Haggard and Hughes, 1991) because of the low yield of important previously unknown losses, and the high incidence of serious otitis media in this group, which would cause the unnecessary referral of large numbers of children with transient losses. It is strongly advocated that parental checklists be used and that concerns about hearing or communication abilities are referred promptly for diagnostic tests. However, it must be recognized that a system which depends upon parental vigilance may be least effective for those children most in need.

Screening test at five years

A pure-tone screening test is given as part of the initial school medical examination. To 'pass', children must make a conditioned response to tones presented to each ear at 20 dB, (or sometimes 25 dB), across the frequency range important for speech perception. Whilst this test does identify children with problems, many feel that the criterion of what is 'acceptable' is insufficiently stringent (Northern and Downs, 1984).

Screening for conductive losses

Because the screening tests described are insufficiently sensitive to identify many conductive losses, it has been suggested that routine **immittance tests** (tympanometry) be included in the screening procedure. The potential advantages are considerable: these tests are 'objective'; they require only the passive cooperation of the child and provide an extremely useful diagnostic assessment of middle ear function independently of the rest of the hearing mechanism. But it is not a test of hearing as such, so must always be used in conjunction with other tests. Immittance testing is an extremely sensitive procedure and unless the limits of 'acceptability' are set very broadly, it may identify far more children as having potential hearing/ear problems than can be dealt with by the system, or than is necessary for their well-being. At present, therefore, its use with babies is more pertinent for those who are already identified as needing further hearing evaluation rather than as part of the initial screening procedure.

DIAGNOSTIC TESTS OF HEARING

Children referred to the audiology clinic for assessment include those considered 'at risk for hearing loss', children who may be 'difficult to test' because of specific problems and those for whom doubt about hearing has been expressed, as well as those who have 'failed' a screening test. It is important that audiology clinics maintain an open referral policy if as many children with hearing impairment as possible are to be identified.

In diagnostic tests of hearing the **procedural aims** are: to confirm or refute the existence of a hearing loss, to establish the level of acuity across the frequency range for each ear separately, to identify the site of lesion and, where possible, to establish the cause. With very young children, the results of one visit are often tentative, unless normal responses are found. A follow-up visit is usually required to confirm initial findings before appropriate action is taken, and management planned.

Tests are carried out in sound-reduced conditions with highly skilled testers. For results to be reliable and valid, a battery of tests must be administered. Initial tests are subjective and evaluate the child's behavioural responses to sound. At present it is considered that these behavioural procedures provide the best indication of total hearing function for most children. Where there are problems and doubts about the reliability of results, some objective tests, which involve the electrical recording of physiological responses to sound, (mentioned below) can provide invaluable corroborative information.

Initially, a screening procedure is repeated, under more stringent control, ensuring that the test method selected is appropriate for the maturational level of the child. If the child fails to respond to the test stimuli at 'minimal' levels (25–35 dB), intensity is progressively raised until a response is elicited. A record is then made of the level of intensity required for response to each of the sound stimuli. In the specialist clinic, a variety of responses may be accepted as a hearing response, although skilled judgement is needed in their interpretation.

Sound stimuli used in 'free-field' testing will include warbled tones (two oscillating tones which are very close in frequency). Children generally find these tones interesting and will respond well to them. Their precise control enables the measurement of the child's response at specific frequencies and intensities. Since some children respond differentially to different sounds, a variety of sounds are normally used to ensure that response levels do reflect hearing acuity rather than lack of interest in the sound. Speech sounds are included: most usually a 'hum' which has exclusively low frequency components and a 's' sound, which, if produced in a specific way, comprises only high frequencies. Although such sounds may be difficult to produce to accurate intensity specification, their inclusion may be important since some babies respond preferentially to voice. To overcome the difficulties, some clinics utilize recorded speech stimuli via loudspeakers so that output may be precisely controlled by an attenuator.

Age-appropriate tests of hearing acuity

Although ages are indicated as a guideline, it is the developmental level of the child rather than his chronological age which determines the choice of test.

6 – 18 months: The 'distraction' test is used, as described earlier.

18 – 30 months: When a child has developed some understanding of simple phrases, these are incorporated into the test to gauge his understanding of speech at measured intensities. Phrases and vocabulary used must be checked first to ensure that they are familiar to the child. A four toy eye-pointing test may be used. Since these measures cannot assess specific frequency response, it is supplemented by a warbled tone distraction test, focusing particularly on high frequencies.

30 – 36 months: At this stage a child is normally able to make a simple conditioned response to the sound stimulus (e.g. he must put a brick in the box when he hears the tone.) Where possible, warbled tones are used. In this way precise levels of threshold response at specific frequencies may be determined. A speech test, (usually a 'toy test') is administered additionally, where possible, to assess speech discrimination abilities at measured intensities. Since the tests described are 'free-field', the separate performance of each ear is not assessed, unless a masker is used to occlude the ear not being tested. An indication of whether both ears have similar thresholds may be gained by assessing the child's ability to localize sound source accurately. These tests provide an indication of total hearing function, and cannot identify site of lesion.

From 3 years: The child may be ready to make a conditioned response to conventional pure tone audiometry, using headphones, which permits threshold measurements for each ear separately. Additionally, tests of bone conduction response can bypass middle ear function and

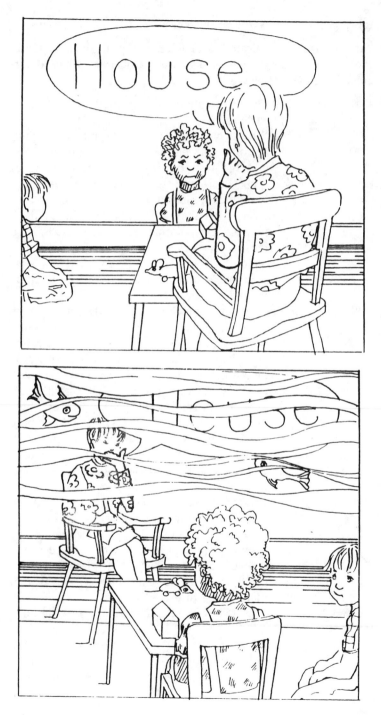

thus indicate whether the loss is conductive or sensori-neural. The results of this test are plotted on an **audiogram**. A speech test (e.g. McCormick 14 toy test) may be given where possible. This assessment will corroborate pure tone test findings as well as providing information about speech discrimination abilities.

In addition to the tests described above, all children will have an otoscopic examination and immittance tests, to assess outer and middle ear status, and thus clarify site of lesion. A history will be taken, normally from the parents; this is seen as an important contribution to the assessment.

In most instances, the procedure outlined will provide a clear picture of the child's hearing abilities, although initial test results are always considered tentative and must be repeated.

Where doubts exist, further tests will be undertaken. These may include 'objective' tests, such as auditory brainstem evoked response measurements (ABR), or recording oto-acoustic emissions. Both these tests are non-invasive and relatively simple to administer. Other tests (e.g. electro-cochleography) are invasive and administered under general anaesthetic.

The choice of additional test will depend upon the needs of the individual and, at present, upon availability of the facilities required. None gives a definitive answer about hearing; final diagnosis will depend upon careful consideration of all the assessment findings.

ROLE OF PARENTS AND PROFESSIONALS IN THE DETECTION OF HEARING PROBLEMS

We have looked at ways in which trained individuals assess hearing at various stages in development. Parents and other professionals who come into contact with the child regularly also have a very significant part to play in the early identification of hearing loss. This regular contact offers ideal opportunities in which to observe the child's pattern of response to environmental sounds and speech, and to note behaviours which may lead to the suspicion of a hearing loss. There are several different kinds of behaviour, of either a transient or long-standing nature, which may indicate the presence of a hearing loss, even in the absence of any clinical signs. However it should be noted that these behaviours also occur in children who hear normally.

Lack of attention. The child in question seems inattentive or unaware of things going on around him. He is not easily alerted to the fact that someone is speaking, or to changes in the environment. He may also have difficulty sustaining attention over a period of time.

Constantly looks at the speaker's face. The child with a stable hearing deficit may develop ingenious compensation strategies. For example, many such children learn (often unconsciously) to pay attention to the speaker's lip movements and facial expressions. This provides them with valuable information to supplement their impaired hearing, and may successfully disguise a hearing loss.

Responds to some sounds. Apparent responses to sound may in fact be responses to other events such as the draught of air (rather than the noise produced) when the door opens. Alternatively, the child may respond to those sounds which are within his audible range. To those who are unaware that a hearing loss may be partial, or in a certain range of frequencies only, this may seem to be proof that the child can hear 'when he wants to'.

Responds inconsistently on different days. The child who seems to respond on some days but not on others may be experiencing an intermittent hearing loss as a result of otitis media. This can be extremely confusing, both for the adult observing this type of behaviour, and for the child. Children with fluctuating hearing losses are often wrongly described as being naughty or wilful, since they behave perfectly normally when their hearing is unimpaired, and at other times, for no apparent reason, seem to switch off from their environment. This may be explained by the fact that at these times their hearing is down, or else that they have developed poor listening habits. There may be no other more obvious reason, such as a cold or a high temperature, to indicate that hearing is affected.

Responds poorly to speech when in noisy surroundings. The child with a slight or moderate hearing loss may respond well in good listening conditions, however in a noisy environment, such as a classroom, or at home with the television on, the level of background noise obscures the spoken message. As a result, the child frequently fails to hear, or mishears instructions, or asks for repetitions. The relationship between this type of behaviour and ambient noise levels may not at first be obvious. Those of us with normal hearing are able to selectively attend to speech and quickly adapt to difficult listening conditions. The masking effects of a noisy environment are far greater when hearing is impaired.

Speech is difficult to understand. When a child's speech is unintelligible, this may be a direct consequence of impaired hearing; if he is unable to perceive all the elements of speech, he must clearly have difficulties in reproducing them accurately. Many such children are also poor at assessing the accuracy of their own speech patterns, which further confounds their intelligibility problems.

Speaks very quietly/loudly. This type of behaviour indicates that the child is not perceiving his own voice normally. The child who speaks very quietly may have a conductive hearing loss, since he can still hear his own voice through bone conduction even though sound reception via air conduction is impaired. The child with a sensori-neural loss, where air and bone conducted sound are equally affected (since the problem is located beyond the middle ear) may speak loudly in order to hear his voice at all.

Speech and understanding are limited. The child with impaired hearing hears less, and receives a degraded message, and so is likely to develop comprehension and use of language more slowly than normal.

Where any of the above behaviours are noted, either singly or in combination, referral for a medical opinion is advisable. An audiological assessment can then be arranged. The involvement of a speech therapist may also be valuable in order to obtain an assessment of the child's level of language development and thereby identify or confirm any suspected problems. Appropriate intervention can then begin.

There may be grounds to suspect an ear infection in a young child with an upper respiratory tract infection, with or without a high temperature, or a child who is irritable and indicates that his ears are a source of pain (perhaps by rubbing them). In these cases, referral for a medical opinion is essential.

WHY KNOWING HELPS: MINIMIZING THE EFFECTS OF A HEARING LOSS

Subsequent management will depend on the outcome of the assessments referred to above. However there are three principal areas to address: medical intervention, provision and use of hearing aids, and developing the use of tactics to facilitate communication.

If a management programme to minimize the effects of a young child's hearing loss is to be successful, the role of parents is crucial. To be effective in this role, they must understand the specific nature and effects of the hearing loss. Without the basis of understanding, parents will not appreciate the reasons for making the small modifications necessary, nor the benefits to be derived. They are, therefore, unlikely to implement suggestions.

Medical and surgical intervention

All children with hearing loss need regular otoscopic examinations. Where the canal is occluded with wax, and the drum cannot be visualized, the wax must be removed before testing continues.

Where the hearing loss is **conductive**, medical intervention will normally be the first consideration. Medical intervention for **otitis media** will aim to eliminate the cause of the problem. Treatment may include antibiotics, cleaning of the ear, and sometimes additional medication such as decongestants. Where such treatment is unsuccessful, and the pathology persists, surgical intervention may be considered. The aim is normally to drain and ventilate the middle ear space, so that the ear remains healthy. Where possible, patency of the Eustachian tubes is restored. **Adenoids** may be removed if they are enlarged and blocking the nasopharyngeal openings to the Eustachian tubes. Where fluid within the middle ear is very thick, it may be aspirated via a tiny hole in the ear drum under anaesthetic. This procedure is known as a **myringotomy**.

Where it proves impossible/inappropriate to restore Eustachian tube patency, middle ear **ventilation tubes** (grommets) may be fitted. These tubes provide a tiny artificial airway to the middle ear through the eardrum, which once more equalizes pressure either side of the drum. If successful, this procedure may restore hearing and health to the middle ears. However, it does not offer a total panacea. Sometimes, tubes require repeated replacement where chronic middle ear problems persist and many specialists are concerned by the damage caused to the eardrum by repeated tube insertion. New procedures and devices currently in use are addressing these difficulties (East, 1986).

As the child approaches adolescence, he develops immunity to many upper respiratory infections. Additionally, with growth, the

Eustachian tubes provide a less efficient pathway for infection to spread to the middle ears. In consequence, hearing difficulties tend to resolve. This fact, the short-lived effects of some surgical procedures and impossibly long hospital waiting lists, have all been used as justification for a delay in intervention. In arriving at this decision, the needs of the individual child and the effects of the hearing loss on his total development must be considered.

Although **sensori-neural losses** are not remediable, a cochlear implant may provide limited but potentially useful information about sound through the insertion of electrodes in the cochlea, which stimulate the auditory nerve directly. This procedure, originally developed for use with adults with acquired hearing losses, is now being used with young, profoundly deaf children who must meet very stringent criteria.

It is extremely important that children with sensori-neural impairment do not have their hearing problems compounded by additional conductive difficulties. An additional loss of acuity of even 10 dB may have a devastating effect on a child already struggling to learn language and cope with the stresses of school. For these children, regular tympanometry and an otoscopic examination provide necessary and adequate surveillance.

Hearing aids: their effective use

Hearing aids are essentially miniature loudspeaker systems – they serve to amplify sound. Since this is generally what is required with a conductive loss, such individuals often do well with hearing aids. However, with advances in middle ear surgery, the number of children and adults wearing hearing aids because of a conductive loss has decreased. Where appropriate, hearing aids may provide much needed amplification, but it is important to realize that even the most sophisticated hearing aids cannot restore normal hearing. With careful use, it is possible to maximize the benefit obtained from hearing aids.

For the individual with a sensori-neural loss, currently available hearing aids are less effective. This is because of the nature of the loss, which is characterized by poor discrimination ability. Simply boosting the intensity of the signal cannot make it sound clearer.

Among the variety of hearing aids available today, the most common are the body-worn aids and the behind-the-ear (postaural) aids. Body-worn aids have several drawbacks: although larger, more robust and easier to manipulate than miniaturized aids, their size makes them cosmetically less attractive. The cords which attach the receiver to the aid are unsightly and easily broken. Finally, since body-worn aids are worn on or under clothing, the effect of clothing rubbing against the microphone can cause a loud and disturbing noise. For these reasons, and rapid advances in miniaturized hearing aid technology, body-worn aids are less widely used now than previously.

Behind-the-ear aids are smaller and easier to conceal than body-worn aids. As they are worn at ear level, sound reception more closely resembles that of the ear. Furthermore, where two aids are worn, there are benefits in sound localization. There are disadvantages related to the small size of the instrument when adjusting controls and inserting batteries. The likelihood of acoustic feedback occurring is increased because all components are housed in such a compact unit. Finally, where children are concerned, they are also easier to lose and more vulnerable to being damaged. However, as they have improved in quality and become more powerful, their popularity and use has increased. (For a fuller account, the section on amplification in Northern and Downs, 1984, is recommended.)

Introduction of hearing aids to a child must be a careful process if the child is to be persuaded to use them to maximum benefit. Unless the parents are sufficiently committed to the hearing aids, the child is likely to pick up any negative feelings and reject the aids. Hearing aids are initially uncomfortable to wear; earmoulds have to be individually made, and even then it may be difficult to achieve the perfect fit. The sound received may seem intrusive and unnatural at first. Where there is initial reluctance towards using the aids, encouraging the child to wear them for short periods of time and gradually extending these periods may be successful.

Controlling the sounds that the child hears during these early stages is also important, so that he is not overwhelmed by a mass of sound which makes little sense. Hearing aids cannot select and amplify only the important sounds – all sounds are amplified equally. This adds to the child's problem the task of discriminating the spoken message from any unnecessary noise. Minimizing background noise as much as possible will improve the situation. This means turning off appliances (televisions, radios, dishwashers, etc.) when communication is essential; closing windows and doors; ensuring that rooms are carpeted and curtained (thereby reducing the amount of echo); ensuring that a number of people are not all talking at once; raising one's voice slightly (but not shouting), and trying to sit or stand reasonably close (within 1 m is ideal) to the child when speaking, as this will have the effect of increasing the intensity of the spoken message above that of the ambient noise.

Since loudness recruitment is commonly associated with sensorineural hearing loss, it is also wise to avoid shouting or making sudden, loud noises (e.g. a loud handclap to gain attention) wherever possible. Apart from the discomfort caused, such high intensities result in the production of distorted signals by hearing aids.

However, where listening conditions are less than ideal, even those with normal hearing compensate by making use of visual information to supplement the impoverished auditory signal (Summerfield, 1983). For individuals wearing hearing aids, this aspect of speech perception is even more important, and so enabling them to see clearly what is being said is helpful. This can be achieved by making sure that the speaker faces the hearing aid wearer and that the latter is attending; that the speaker's face is well illuminated (i.e. facing, rather than having one's back to a light source); that the speaker's mouth is not obscured or partially covered (e.g. by a hand); that lip patterns are as normal as possible – not distorted by shouting, mumbling or chewing – and that the speaker uses normal gesture and facial expression to help convey the message.

In educational settings, where the acoustic environment falls far short of the requirements needed to use personal hearing aids effectively, special amplification systems are available. An example of one such system is the radio amplification system; here, the child wears a receiver which picks up sound directly from the teacher's microphone via radio waves. This allows the teacher to communicate directly with the child while moving freely around the classroom. Of course, even with systems such as this, the need to get the child's attention and speak whilst facing him/her etc. still apply. The teacher must also remember to turn off the microphone when talking to another child, otherwise the hearing-impaired child is forced to 'listen in', causing unnecessary confusion.

Where the above guidelines are closely observed, hearing aids can provide an essential channel of communication with a hearing-impaired child. However, for most children, the effects of impaired hearing have had some impact by the time hearing aids are provided, and so other management strategies must be implemented concurrently.

An effective way to minimize the disadvantage of children with any degree of hearing impairment is to modify their listening and language-learning environment and help them to develop compensatory strategies. The approaches discussed later, in Chapter 8 are also of relevance here.

TACTICS TO FACILITATE COMMUNICATION

Ways of improving the listening environment and making the most of visual cues have been mentioned in the previous section. In addition, small changes in the approach to communication with hearing impaired children can be highly effective.

Children with a relatively small hearing loss are frequently described as 'not bothering to listen', 'tuning out of the conversation', 'uninterested.' This does not reflect their lack of desire to communicate, but merely that communication can be difficult for them. The process can be simplified by ensuring that the child is made aware of the context of the conversation (by stating the topic of conversation, or using a gesture to indicate what is being discussed, for example), thereby making language more predictable.

The complexity of language used must be appropriate to the child's level of understanding. Parents and others need to be aware of the complexity of their own language, to recognize vocabulary and expressions which are not known to the child and be ready to explain or clarify as necessary.

Hearing impaired children may not indicate that they are failing to understand. Instead, they may respond by guessing, by giving neutral or negative responses, or by withdrawing from the communication situation altogether. They must learn to identify situations where their understanding is incomplete, and be encouraged to ask for clarification. It is equally important for parents and others to indicate when they have not understood what the child has said. The child can then be encouraged to rephrase and, where necessary, use gesture to make the meaning clear.

Above all, the child must be an equal partner in conversation and feel that their contribution is valued. Studies have indicated that in situations where adults dominate conversations with children, the children's contributions are reduced (Wood *et al.*, 1986).

Case study 5.1

Aisha, aged four years five months, from an English Punjabi family, was referred for speech therapy after a routine developmental check showed her to have very little intelligible speech and probable learning difficulties.

Initial speech therapy assessment indicated that Aisha failed to respond to speech unless intensity was raised considerably, when her understanding of English and of Punjabi was at the level of a two-year-old. Although Aisha's speech was largely not understood at home, it was found that the apparent jargon was meaningful, well-intonated English phrases which incorporated some Punjabi.

Audiological tests indicated impacted wax in both canals, 'glue ears', and a bilateral loss of 40–60 dB across the frequency range. Her ears were syringed and she was placed on the waiting list for myringotomy and insertion of grommets. Speech therapy incorporating parent guidance was instigated. Progress was rapid; surgery three months later greatly improved her hearing. When she started mainstream school at five, her speech was mainly intelligible and her understanding of language was near that of a four-year-old.

Once in school, Aisha's reading skills developed rapidly, but in class she failed to participate in most group activities. It was reported that her attention was poor and that she abandoned tasks easily. Appointments for follow-up hearing checks and speech therapy were not kept because her mother was now working full-time. At 5 years 7 months Aisha's teacher was concerned that she was wrongly placed in a mainstream class.

Case study 5.2

Maria, aged five years nine months was reported to be experiencing difficulties at primary school. Her teacher described her as 'rather immature and impulsive; speech is sometimes indistinct; seems to be of average intelligence'. The fourth of five children, her family described her as a quiet child, who was not always attentive and at times seemed to be in 'a world of her own'.

From her records it was noted that she had passed infant hearing screening, but had failed pure tone testing at school entry. Following referral for further testing, she was diagnosed as having a marked high frequency sensori-neural loss, possibly of insidious onset.

Maria was transferred to a hearing impaired unit school and was provided with two hearing aids. She immediately seemed to be more responsive in one-to-one situations, although she did not like wearing aids in the classroom.

Speech therapy assessment showed her to have systematic problems with discrimination and production of high frequency consonants, e.g. 's', 'sh'. Her understanding of language was below what would be expected for her age. In addition, her vocabulary was felt to be limited and she made frequent errors with use of grammatical word endings. A course of speech therapy was initiated, following which her ability to discriminate and produce high frequency consonants improved, although she had difficulty in integrating these sounds into everyday speech. Her language skills progressed steadily; however, a year later they were still delayed.

Case study 5.3

Leroy, aged three years ten months, was referred for speech therapy assessment from the ENT clinic which he attended because of recurrent bouts of otitis media and a fluctuating hearing loss of 35–45 dB over the previous two years. His parents were aware that his hearing fluctuated, but did not feel that it posed any problems.

On assessment, he presented as a friendly, talkative child who co-operated well with formal testing. Both his understanding and expressive language proved to be age appropriate. His parents were intuitively providing a good language environment which took into consideration his changing hearing levels. No speech therapy intervention was indicated, but since he was about to start at nursery, arrangements were made to meet with the teacher to ensure his hearing needs were known and appropriately managed.

SUMMARY AND CONCLUSIONS

It is possible to extract the following points from the preceeding discussion.

- There are essentially two different types of hearing loss – sensori-neural and conductive. The former is generally more pervasive than the latter but the latter is much more common.

- What constitutes a significant hearing loss remains unclear. The 25 dB loss recognized as a cut-off for adults is not normally thought to be adequately sensitive for children when they are first learning language.
- Hearing loss is likely to have a profound effect on the child's social and educational life. These problems are multiplied if the loss coincides with other difficulties.
- A variety of procedures are available for screening hearing in young children. Discussion continues as to whether such procedures are sufficiently accurate for universal application.
- Parents provide essential information in the identification process.
- There are a variety of ways of improving the child's ability to benefit from the auditory environment.

A hearing loss has been described as 'an irreversible learning disaster'. This pessimistic description reflects society's lack of flexibility in recognizing ways around the problem, rather than a description of the disability. Texts which discuss the effects of deafness on language and general development emphasize that the extent of the hearing loss is only one of many variables which may influence the child's performance.

A hearing impaired child is, potentially, a normal communicator. The nature and extent of his hearing loss must be identified early and appropriate management implemented if this potential is to be realized. Provided that parents and teachers recognize the role of hearing, both in language and general development, they can be successful in minimizing the deficits and, where necessary, in devising alternative approaches.

The examination of hearing should be seen as an integral part of the study of the early identification of language impairment. Although the two interact in a variety of ways it is impossible to judge one without an effective evaluation of the other.

REFERENCES

Balkany, T. J. (1980) Otologic aspects of Down's syndrome. *Seminars in Speech Language and Hearing*, **1**, 39.

Bennett, M. J. (1975) The auditory response cradle: a device for the objective assessment of auditory state in the neonate. *Symposium Zoological Society*, **37**, 291–305.

Bess, F. H. (1982) Children with unilateral hearing loss. *Journal of Academy of Rehabilitation Audiology*, **15**, 131–144.

Bishop, D. V. M. and Edmundson, A. (1986) Is otitis media a major cause of specific developmental language disorders? *British Journal of Disorders of Communication*, **21**, 321–338.

Bluestone, C. D. and Shurin, P. A. (1974) Middle ear disease in childhood: pathogenesis, diagnosis and management. *Paediatric Clinics of North America*, **21**, 379–400.

Dobie, R. A., and Berlin, C. I. (1979) Influence of otitis media on hearing and development. *Annals of Otology Rhinology & Laryngology*, **88** (2) (suppl. 60), 48–53.

Downs, M. P. (1980) Communication disorders in Down's syndrome. *Seminars in Speech Language and Hearing*, **1**, 1.

East, D. (1986) The use of Per-Lee ventilation tubes in the management of refractory secretory otitis media. *The Journal of Laryngology*, **100**, 509–513.

Haggard, M. P. and Hughes, E. (1991) *Screening Children's Hearing: A review of the literature and implications of otitis media*, HMSO, London.

Hall, D. M. B. (Ed.) (1989) Health For All Children, Oxford Medical Publications, Oxford.

Hitchings, V. and Haggard, M. P. (1983) Incorporation of parental suspicion in screening infants' hearing. *British Journal of Audiology*, **17**, 71–76.

Jerger, S., Jerger, J., Alford, B. R. and Abrams, S. (1983) Development of speech intelligibility in children with recurrent otitis media. *Ear & Hearing*, **4**, 138–145.

McCormick, B. (1988) *Screening for Hearing Impairment in Young Children*, Croom Helm, London.

Northern, J. L. and Downs, M. P. (1984) *Hearing in Children*, 3rd edn, Williams & Wilkins, Baltimore.

Simmons, F. B. and Russ, F. N. (1974) Automated newborn screening: the cribogram. *Archives of Laryngology*, **100**, 1–7.

Stevens, J. C. *et al.* (1987) A comparison of otoacoustic emissions and brainstem electric response audiometry in the normal newborn and babies admitted to a special care baby unit. *Clinical Physics and Physiological Measurements*, **8**, 95–104.

Summerfield, A. Q. (1983) Audiovisual speech perception, lipreading and artificial simulation, in *Hearing Science and Hearing Disorders*, (eds M. E. Lutman and M. P. Haggard), Academic Press, London, pp. 132–182.

Teele, D. W., Klein, J. O. and Rosner, B. (1980) Epidemiology of otitis media in children. *Annals of Otology Rhinology Laryngology*, **89**, (suppl. 68), 5–60.

Tucker, S. M. (1986) Auditory screening of normal and preterm infants using the auditory response cradle. *Audiology in practice* II, 45–47.

Wood, D., Wood, H., Griffiths, A. and Howarth, I. (1986) *Teaching and Talking with Deaf Children*, John Wiley, Chichester.

6

The process of early identification

James Law

Considerable time and energy has been devoted both to designing and to carrying out a wide variety of procedures for identifying children with language impairment. This chapter begins by discussing the relative meaning of the terms 'examination', 'surveillance' and 'screening'. It then turns to identifying the criteria which should be used to evaluate all screening measures and a wide variety of such measures are examined. Finally the chapter will turn to the subject of who should carry out identification procedures and which ages are most appropriate for doing so.

IS LANGUAGE SCREENING 'SCREENING'?

Screening often appears to be a relatively straightforward concept, that is a means of checking whether someone does or does not have a problem. As we have seen in Chapter 2, the difficulty arises when we try to specify what a language impairment entails. There has been some discussion recently as to whether 'screening' is a suitable description of the process (Hall, 1989). The potential confusion arises, in part, from the need for those involved in such processes to share a common terminology when describing the process. There are at least three commonly used terms which need to be considered.

1. Screening
2. Examining
3. Surveillance.

Screening

One of the most widely accepted definitions of screening has been given by the American Committee on Chronic Illness (1957):

... the presumptive identification of unrecognised disease or defect by the application of tests, examinations and other procedures, which can be applied rapidly (to) sort out apparently well persons who may have a disease from those that probably do not.

Cochrane and Holland (1971) stipulate six widely accepted conditions which must be met if a screening test is to be described as such.

1. Easy and quick to administer.
2. Acceptable to subjects.
3. Accurate in measuring any attribute being tested.
4. Precise, giving consistent results in the hands of different testers.
5. Sensitive in the hands of different testers.
6. Specific, giving a high percentage of negative results when the subjects do not have the disease.

As the use of the term 'disease' suggests, the term 'screening' carries distinctly medical connotations. It is important to understand that the term is conventionally used for clearly defined medical conditions such as phenylketonuria, and although its use has spread into developmental paediatrics it has done so rather uneasily.

A number of authors have expressed reservations about the term 'screening'. Court (1976) for example dismissed the use of the term completely as being inappropriate for all but a handful of very specific cases, Whitmore and Bax (1988) maintain that it is not suitable for any complex behaviours, amongst which language is an obvious example. Hall (1989) similarly feels that the term should be discarded for all but the most specific measures. He maintains that for many conditions there is insufficient agreement as to what is and what is not a clinical case. He uses this argument to suggest reducing the extent to which primary health care professionals in the UK actively look for cases.

Examining

In their paper 'Screening or Examining', Whitmore and Bax (1988) point out that the American Commission on Chronic Illness only advocated the use of screening as a substitute for routine clinical examination at a time of shortage of medical manpower. They distinguish between screening for PKU as a specific and preventable cause of mental handicap and identifying develop-mental delay of an uncertain aetiology. In other words there is a difference between looking for disease and anticipating disability. They accept the need to search for cases of children with disability, but are convinced that the measures which are used should not be construed as screens at all. Rather they should be seen as a part of the overall examination.

Surveillance

In the report 'Fit for the Future' Court (1976) rejected 'the very notion of a developmental screening programme'. Instead the report advocated a programme of 'health surveillance'. Whitmore and Bax take issue with this use of terminology maintaining that 'surveillance' actually means to watch or guard over a suspected person, prisoner, or the like, suggesting the very paternalism which the health service was trying to discard at the time.

We are left with the term 'screening' being commonly used as a term to describe the process of looking for cases in whatever form it may take. Unfortunately this very loose use of the term is, in the end, rather unhelpful. There is a clear distinction between one professional actively assessing a child's abilities and another talking to a parent in the street in an informal fashion and making a clinical judgement as to whether a child needs to be referred on.

In the light of the discussion above it is justifiable to retain the term 'screening test' for any test which has been developed within the framework outlined by Cochrane and Holland (1971) but it should be discarded unless these conditions have been met. Clearly the term 'screening' is inappropriate as a generic term for any procedures which helps the doctor or health visitor to pick out new cases. For this reason 'early identification procedures' is recommended.

THE EVALUATION OF PROCEDURES

Given the resources and energy allocated to running early identi-fication programmes it is important that they are monitored as closely as possible. To a certain extent, of course, if the staff administering them and those receiving the referrals are happy with the procedure then it can be said to work. However it is often necessary to show others that the procedures are effective by demonstrating both that the children who are identified are correctly targetted and that those that are not identified have not been missed. It is rare of course that any procedure will have a one hundred per cent success rate. So evaluation often becomes a discussion about levels of acceptability. There are two basic concepts – **validity** and **reliability** – which need to be borne in mind when developing any screening procedure.

Validity

Face validity

Face validity refers to a wide clinical acceptance that the skills to be examined are indeed relevant. This would normally be derived from an examination of the relevant literature but it could equally well come from a consensus amongst those involved in generating the measure.

Construct validity

Construct validity refers to the extent to which the structure of the test itself affects the test's capacity to reflect the performance criterion. This might be a function of the training offered to those using the measure. Thus great care needs to be taken in administering the test. Clearly if no introduction is given to the materials it is likely to hinder the child's performance. Conversely if care is not taken to avoid eye pointing or indicating non-verbally what is required the child's performance may be unrepresentative of his abilities. Equally it might be a function of the test itself. If the measure is constructed so that more complex tasks are elicited first, the chances of a child preserving to the end are reduced. If the materials used to elicit responses are too developmentally advanced or culturally inappropriate this too will affect construct validity.

Criterion validity

Criterion validity refers to the extent to which the results of the screening measure concerned reflect the performance criterion. In the case of early language screening this means the extent to which the test captures the child's communication skills. In practice this is often accomplished by comparing the child's screen score to performance on a recognized assessment of the same ability. Such an assessment is termed the **gold standard.**

The relationship between the screen and the gold standard can then be expressed as follows:

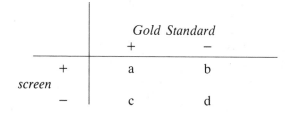

This, then allows us to examine specificity and sensitivity.

A specific test is one that identifies the true negatives correctly (Barker and Rose, 1984). So a screen is said to be specific if those that fail the screen are correctly identified. Thus the number of false positives is acceptably low. Normally this would be measured by a predetermined assessment or specific set of predetermined and easily recognizable criteria. This can be expressed as an equation as follows:

$$\text{Specificity} = \text{True Negatives}/(\text{False positives} + \text{True negatives})$$
$$\text{or } d/b+d$$

Sensitivity refers to a test's ability to detect a high proportion of true cases (Barker and Rose, 1984). A screen can be said to be sensitive if those that pass the screen do not turn out to have problems. Thus the number of false negatives is acceptably low. The same process for monitoring this would be adopted as it would for specificity. This can be expressed as an equation as follows:

$$\text{Sensitivity} = \text{True Positives}/(\text{False negatives} + \text{True positives})$$
$$\text{or } a/c+a$$

In general there is less information available about the sensitivity than the specificity of measures developed. On the one hand those developing screens are usually more interested in those identified, and on the other it is an extremely expensive exercise to look for children who have been missed.

In addition to its specificity and sensitivity any screening test can also be evaluated in terms of its ability to predict a positive or negative result. A positive result can be predicted by $a/a+b$, which allows us to calculate the likelihood of a person with language impairment really having such a difficulty. Similarly, the likelihood of a negative result is d/c+d.

It is also possible to speak of a test predicting subsequent performance. Prediction of subsequent behaviour is a daunting task and it often seems rather unrealistic to expect a short measure at a specific point in time to pick out children who will have persistent language problems (see Stevenson, 1984). Yet the fact remains that, as we saw in Chapter 2, one of the great unanswered questions in speech pathology is how to differentiate between children who will go on to have difficulties and those who will improve spontaneously. So, in the development of any screening protocol, an attempt should be made to measure the efficacy of the process of identification at two points in time.

Reliability

Screening is essentially a practical exercise. For it to work it must be possible for those involved to achieve repeatable results. Two types of 'repeatability' or reliability are identified.

Inter-tester reliability

Inter-tester reliability is the ability of two testers to achieve the same results on the same test over an acceptably short period of time.

Intra-tester reliability

Intra-tester reliability is the ability of the same tester to repeat results on a single measure.

Reliability should not be confused with validity because as Plewis and Bax (1982) have pointed out, just because a procedure is reliable does not mean that it is also valid. Having said that, the reverse probably is true. An unreliable test is unlikely to be valid. Two potential complications which permeate all measurement of children's language need to be borne in mind. Children may perform differently from day to day. Care will need to be taken that conditions are optimal for any such assessment. Similarly the nature of development is such that the time period between assessment and reassessment should be minimal to avoid the possibility of language change in the intervening period.

TYPES OF ASSESSMENT

To date, no real attempt has been made to classify the various screening procedures that have been produced. This is probably in part because of the potential confusion inherent in doing so. Many of the assessments do not readily lend themselves to comparison. Nevertheless there are two principal types; **multiphasic** and **monophasic**. The second of the two may be further subdivided into two groups; **primary** and **diagnostic**. A number of such tests are reviewed below to give readers a flavour of the range of material available.

Multiphasic tests

Multiphasic tests are those designed to assess all aspects of children's development throughout their early years.

1. The Denver Developmental Screen Test

- (Frankenburg *et al.*, 1967, 1971; Bryant *et al.*, 1974; Meisels, 1989; Borowitz and Glascoe, 1986)
- Age range: 2 weeks to 6 years 4 months
- Behaviours tested: Personal–social, fine motor-adaptive, language, gross motor
- Materials: Eight specific objects and a test with 105 test items
- Number of children on which it was developed: 1036
- Results: 'Co-positivity' of 0.73, 'co-negativity' of 0.92; 7.2% over-referral and 2.95% under-referral (Frankenburg and Dodds, 1967); 'co-positivity' of 0.92, 'co-negativity' of 0.97; 3.2% over-referral and 0.4% under-referral (Frankenburg *et al.*, 1971)
- Criterion: Stanford Binet, Revised Bayley Scale of Infant Development (Frankenburg *et al.*, 1967, 1971)
- Comment: Bryant *et al.* (1974) found that children from Cardiff, UK, performed differently from Denver children on both gross motor and language scales. In reviewing more than a dozen studies, Meisels (1989) found that, although the test is highly specific in that it does not miss children, it has unacceptably low sensitivity. In other words it will miss children who are developmentally delayed. He quotes one study in which a five-year-old using two word utterances and with a severe articulation problem was considered to be within the normal range (Borowitz and Glascoe, 1989). This same study indicated that 47% of children with delayed

expressive language were not identified using the Denver Developmental Screening Test. Despite these misgivings it remains the most widely used procedure in the US and indeed throughout the world.

2. The Minnesota Child Development Inventory

- (Ireton and Thwing, 1976; Ireton *et al.*, 1977; Sturner *et al.*, 1982; Gottfried *et al.*, 1984)
- Age range: 2 months to 6 years
- Behaviours tested: General development, gross motor, fine motor, expressive language, comprehension–conceptual, situation comprehension, self-help, personal–social
- Materials: A booklet with 320 items to which the mother responds yes or no, as appropriate
- Number of children on which it was developed: Initially 796 (Ireton and Thwing, 1976); subsequently 109 (Ireton *et al.*, 1977); shortened version (Sturner *et al.*, 1982), 382; study looking at predictive ability (Gottfried *et al.*, 1984), 89–98 at 30/36 and 42 months
- Results: (Sturner *et al.*, 1982) sensitivity of 0.63 and specificity of 0.81, high number of omitted responses in low SES group; (Gottfried *et al.*, 1984) sensitivity of 0.8 and specificity of 0.97, reasonable predictive ability reported in all but motor skills
- Criterion: Stanford Binet (Sturner *et al.*, 1982); McCarthy (Gottfried *et al.*, 1984)
- Comment: Very easy to administer although there is some indication that self-administration resulted in over-referral of group of lower socio-economic status.

3. Schedule for Growing Skills

- (Bellman *et al.*, 1985; Bellman and Cash, 1985)
- Age range: Originally 0–3 years, subsequently 0–5 years
- Behaviours tested: Posture and large movements, vision and fine movements, hearing and speech, social behaviour and play
- Materials: Originally the child's own toys. Subsequently a specific set of toys
- Number of children on which it was developed: 25 for validity, 20 for reliability (Bellman *et al.*, 1985)
- Results: Sensitivity 0.44–0.82, specificity 0.94–1.0, reliability 40% complete agreement, 80% agreement within three months

- Criterion: Griffiths Mental Development Scales (Griffiths, 1970)
- Comment: Comparatively little evaluation beyond the initial study. No evidence of evaluation of scale extended through from three years to five years or the completely new language scale.

Monophasic tests

Monophasic tests are those intended to target a specific behaviour – in this case speech and/or language.

a – Primary Screening Tests

These are administered by primary health care workers at the initial point of contact with the child and parent. This will be in the child health clinic, the general practitioner's or in the US the paediatrician's surgery.

1. The Surrey Speech Screening Test
- (Radway and Norfolk, 1971)
- Age range: 4 years 9 months to 5 years 6 months
- Behaviours tested: Consonants in single words
- Materials: A set of twelve coloured pictures
- Number of children on which it was developed: 783
- Results: 9% requiring treatment; 9.7% requiring observation; 1.7% inappropriately referred (false negatives)
- Criterion: A speech therapist's assessment
- Comment: A simple test. Would probably be considered inadequate in the context of currently accepted linguistic models.

The fact that no 'language' component was included may result in children being referred who are likely to improve spontaneously.

2. Clinical Linguistic and Auditory Milestone Scale
- (Capute and Accardo, 1978; Capute et al., 1986)
- Age range: 0–2 years
- Behaviours tested: Parental report of milestones
- Materials: No materials as such but a style of questioning is specified
- Number of children on which it was developed: 448 (Capute et al., 1986)

- Results: High correlation between 24 of 25 items on the milestone scale and subsequent cognitive performance
- Criterion: Bayley Scales of Infant Development (Bayley, 1969)
- Comment: Raises the question of the reliability of retrospective reporting of milestones. The fact that it only goes up to two years is probably a strength in this respect. The predictive validity would be very interesting given how young the children are when seen.

3. The Early Language Milestone Scale
- (Coplan, 1983; Coplan et al., 1982; Walker et al., 1989)
- Age range: 0–3 years
- Behaviours tested: Parental report of milestones
- Materials: Predominantly questioning of parents, occasional direct elicitation of behaviour from child
- Number of children on which it was developed: 119 (Coplan et al., 1982); 657 (Walker et al., 1989)
- Results: Sensitivity of 97% and specificity of 93% in the initial sample, 87% and 70% in Walker et al., 1989. Very low correspondence between the ELM and the criterion test in the lowest age band
- Criterion: The Sequenced Inventory of Communication Development (Hedrick and Prather, 1984)
- Comment: Appears very sound. It is probably most useful after one year. The same comments pertain to the ELM as they do to the previous scale.

4. The Rigby and Chesham Test
- (Rigby and Chesham, 1981)
- Age range: 4 years 6 months to 4 years 9 months
- Behaviours tested: Speech sounds in isolation and in a spontaneous sentence
- Materials: 12 different objects
- Number of children on whom it was developed: 438
- Results: 14% referred, 2.4% false negatives, 41.9% false positives
- Criterion: Renfrew (Renfrew, 1968) Reynell Developmental Language Scales (Reynell and Huntley, 1985) Edinburgh Articulation Test (Anthony et al., 1971) carried out independently by a speech therapist
- Comment: Similar to the Surrey speech screening test. Very high false positive rate would suggest that this test would

result in extensive over-referral and would therefore be uneconomic.

5. The Levett Muir Language Screening Test
- (Levett and Muir, 1983)
- Age range: 2 years 9 months to 3 years 3 months
- Behaviours tested: Expression, comprehension and phonology
- Materials: A kit involving miniature toys and complex pictures
- Number of children on which it was developed: 1/10 sample of 140 children tested
- Results: 100% agreement on those identified
- Criterion: Reynell Developmental Language Scales (Reynell and Huntley, 1985)
- Comment: Difficult to comment given the very small sample used in the evaluation. The use of the miniatures may make it hard to interpret what it is that the child who does not pass the test finds difficult. This is used in four separate districts in the UK making it the single most popular test for this age group.

6. The Screening Kit of Language Development
- (Bliss and Allen, 1984)
- Age range: 3 years 1 month to 4 years
- Behaviours tested: Vocabulary comprehension, story completion, sentence comprehension, paired sentence repetition with pictures, individual sentence repetition without pictures, auditory comprehension of commands
- Materials: Pictures
- Number of children on which it was developed: 602
- Results: Sensitivity ranged from 0.87 to 1 across the subtests. Specificity ranged from 0.77 to 0.97 across the subtests; somewhat lower figures registered for children using Black American English. Pre-set reliability of 0.85 reached
- Criterion: Sequenced Inventory of Communication Development (Hedrick *et al.*, 1984)
- Comment: A very well-developed test. Although the authors claim that it is a very quick test to administer it is debatable whether the medical staff carrying it out would need such detail to make a referral.

7. The Hackney Early Language Screening Test
- (Dixon *et al.*, 1988; Law, 1991)

- Age range: 2 years 9 months to 3 years
- Behaviours tested: Comprehension and expression
- Materials: Toys and pictures
- Number of children on which it was developed: 40 and then 189
- Results: Sensitivity of 0.98, specificity 0.74. Reliability needs further development
- Criterion: −1.5 standard deviations on the Reynell Developmental Language Scales
- Comment: A very simple test to administer. Shown to be valuable for health visitors. Developed in an inner city area.

8. The Language Development Survey
- (Rescorla, 1989)
- Age range: 2 years
- Behaviours tested: Expressive vocabulary
- Materials: A vocabulary checklist for parents to fill in
- Number of children on which it was developed: 641 in various settings

- Results:

	Delay 1	Delay 2	Delay 3
Sensitivity:	0.53	0.76	0.89
Specificity:	0.97	0.89	0.86

Test/retest reliability = 0.99

- Criterion: Delay 1 = <30 words and no word combinations; Delay 2 = <30 words or no word combinations; Delay 3 = <50 words or no word combinations. These levels were compared to a cut off of six months delay on the expressive scale of the Reynell Developmental Language Scales (Reynell and Huntley, 1985)
- Comment: A very simple test to administer. No problems noted from the effects of parental literacy. Again given how young the children were when seen it would be particularly interesting to see the predictive validity of this measure. Low cut-off rate suggests over-referral is likely.

9. MacArthur Communicative Development Inventories
- (Fenson et al., 1991; Dale, 1991)
- Age range: CDI/Infants 8–16 months; CDI/Toddlers 16–30 months
- Behaviours tested: CDI/Infants words understood and used; CDI/Toddlers words used + morphological/syntactic development + pronominal style
- Material: A form filled in by parents

- Number of children on which it was developed: 1685 in New Haven, Seattle and San Diego in the US
- Test/retest reliability: Not measured
- Criterion: None specified because the project (Fenson *et al.*, 1991) was principally interested in the distribution of performance across a population. Dale (1991) indicates high correlations between CDI/toddler scale with vocabulary test, a high correlation between measures of syntactic complexity (0.76) and MLU. Measurement of pronominal style was not reliable (-0.43)
- Comment: A very simple test to administer. Study population was of above average education. At present care would need to be taken in assuming validity in less-privileged groups. Again figures for predictive validity will be interesting.

b – Diagnostic Screening Tests

These do not fit the conventional definition of screening tests at all. They allow the professional to whom the child is referred to identify levels of competence or to separate out strengths and weaknesses in the child concerned. It is assumed at this stage that the child needs intervention.

1. The Northwestern Syntax Screening Test
- (Lee, 1971)
- Age range: 3 years to 7 years 11 months
- Behaviours tested: Receptive and expressive use of syntax
- Materials: Testing booklet
- Number of children on which it was developed: 344
- Results: Norms are given but no measure of validity or reliability
- Criterion: All children scoring below -2 standard deviations to be treated. all children below the 10th percentile line should be considered for treatment
- Comments: It is acknowledged that great care has to be taken in using the test with children not using the standard American dialect.

2. The Fluharty Preschool Speech and Language Screening Test
- (Fluharty, 1974; Simmons, 1988)
- Age range: 3–5 years
- Behaviours tested: Vocabulary, articulation, receptive language, expressive language

- Materials: A set of 15 objects and pictures
- Number of children on which it was developed: 203 (Fluharty, 1974), 260 (Simmons, 1988)
- Results: Correlation coefficient of validity 0.87, reliability 0.87–1.0 across scales (Fluharty, 1974)
- Criterion: Peabody Picture Vocabulary Test, Goldman Fristoe Test of Articulation, Northwestern Syntax Screening Test
- Comment: Simmons (1988) questions the usefulness of many test items. Often alluded to in the research literature.

3. The Derbyshire Language Rapid Screening Test
- (Masidlover and Knowles, 1982)
- Age range: Not specified but covers preschool language abilities
- Behaviours tested: Comprehension and expression
- Materials: Common toys and pictures
- Number of children on which it was developed: Not specified
- Results: No standardization
- Criterion: None
- Comment: The 'rapid screening test' from the Derbyshire Language Scheme is a part of an integrated programme for children with special needs. Children once assessed are further examined on a more focal 'detailed test of comprehension' which in its turn is cross-referenced with specific teaching activities. Some very rough norms are given based on literature. The authors stress that the scheme is intended for children with learning difficulties for whom the sequence of development is important but for whom age-equivalent levels have little meaning.

4. The Cambridge Screening Test
- (Shahzade et al., 1984)
- Age range: 4 years 5 months to 6 years 2 months
- Behaviours tested: Articulation, discrimination, vocabulary, association/categorization, object function, action/agent, colour concepts, number concepts, commands/spatial relations, memory for commands, digit repetition, diadochokinesis, story sequencing, pragmatic ability
- Materials: Testing booklet, screener's manual, ten coloured cubes
- Number of children on which it was developed: Not specified

- Results: Field tested over two years in Cambridge, Massachusetts, otherwise no further information. Test items are derived from research in developmental psychology and correspond to a variety of different levels
- Criterion: None specified. It is recommended that children scoring 0 on any test item be referred. Score sheets are linked to a class profile
- Comment: A very straightforward, well packaged test. It would be useful for comparing children within a class although difficult to know what to make of the results. Not sufficiently well evaluated to allow comparison with the population of children and too little detail to allow for a full comparison between individuals.

IS THERE AN OPTIMUM FORMAT FOR SCREENING PROCEDURES?

As we have seen above, a variety of different formal procedures have been generated to identify children with speech and language impairment. They are basically of four types.

1. Assessment
2. Checklist
3. Observations
4. A combination

Technically any one of these approaches can be carried out by parent or professional. In practice, assessments have only been used by professionals while checklists and observations have tended to be shared between professionals and parents. Each approach has advantages and disadvantages. So, for example, the assessment approach allows direct observation of the child's elicited performance. Yet as anyone working with preschool children knows all too well they can be unpredictable and simply not perform. If this occurs more commonly with one test rather than a second it must raise questions as to the usefulness of the test in question. In fact in most cases reliability is likely to be more a function of the techniques used to elicit the child's language skills and thus of the training given to those who will be carrying out the test.

The checklist approach is quick and easy to administer. The list may be filled in by parent or professional. In both cases care has to be taken to show clearly what is needed. The more complex the question and the wider the range of options the more likely that the results will be unreliable. Care must be taken that the results are not a function of the literacy of the parent reading the form. Checklists of specific vocabulary items may be a particularly useful approach for the younger child but after the age of two or two-and-a-half it will be too large in most cases for a checklist to be useful. Milestones may similarly be an appropriate subject for a checklist in the early years but, as Hart, Bax and Jenkins (1978)

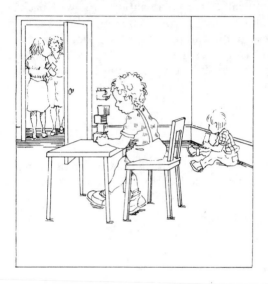

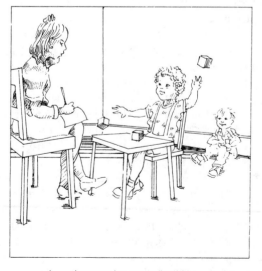

' . . . they can be unpredictable . . . '

have pointed out, the further away the child is from achieving the milestone in question the less likely it is to be accurately reported.

The reliance on observations is likely to be the most commonly used simply because as medical staff become familiar with language development they will be more likely to know what they are looking for. Morever they may know the families concerned and have had a variety of different opportunities to watch the child in the context of his or her family. It has the advantage both of avoiding the formality of testing procedures – carrying necessary equipment around, etc. – and of encouraging those concerned to develop their observational skills, incorporating new findings from developmental psychology and other disciplines in a very immediate fashion. The weakness of this approach is that it is necessary to monitor those children who are referred against a valid benchmark. The dangers with this type of referral system are that it relies too heavily on the idiosyncracies of the observer and makes cross comparison between health districts virtually impossible. The same sort of comment may be made where a combination of approaches is used. Obviously observations are being made all the time but as soon as they are used to extrapolate beyond the measures adopted it becomes very difficult to know what standard is being used.

A combination of testing, the use of checklists and observation probably most accurately reflects the approach used by many primary health workers (see Law, 1991 for a review of approaches currently in use in the UK). They may try one or two activities with the child, ask a few questions and relate what they see to their experience. The difficulty comes in evaluating this as a procedure which others can use. By contrast, although the evaluation of a single procedure is more straightforward it may be difficult to determine where the child's difficulties lie.

THE ROLE OF PARENTS

Given that, as a rule, parents know their children better than any professional is ever likely to do, why do we simply not hand over the responsibility for early identification to them? To do so would certainly save those involved with working with children a lot of effort and resources. Unfortunately, we simply do not know whether parents and professionals share the same expectations of child development.

Miller (1988) has examined the literature relating to parental beliefs about their children's cognitive development. He showed that there is a relationship between parental beliefs about development, their child-rearing practices and their children's development itself. The relationship is clearly complex and it would be wrong to assume causality. Nevertheless the evidence does suggest that parents with low expectations of their children's development are likely to have children who underperform. Although the paper does not concern itself specifically with language development there seems little reason to assume that the same relationship would not hold. Stokes (1991) has reported on a project to compare the results of a test given by nurses and a parent questionnaire with a 'gold standard' test of the type discussed previously. She found that the rates of specificity and sensitivity were comparable for the two approaches at the point at which they were carried out. The principal difference between the two was that the nurses' test had a much stronger predictive ability than the parent questionnaire (82% as against 57%).

We are left, then, with something of a dilemma. On the one hand there is a clear move now towards encouraging parents to become involved in the process of identifying children (see Chapter 7). In many districts in the UK parents are actively encouraged by means of health education literature to comment on their children's speech and language. There have also been videos made specifically to draw parent's attention to the issues involved (Law, 1990). Some authors (Hall, 1989) have even suggested that the onus be placed entirely on the parents to express their anxieties rather than any process by which professionals are actively looking out for cases. Such an approach is in line with the desire to give parents the responsibility for observing their children's development, taking it out of the hands of experts. This has obvious advantages both in terms of the central role it offers the parent and in terms of the opportunity it affords to cut resources allocated to surveillance programmes.

On the other hand, although such a democratic approach would be welcomed by most parents, it is uncertain whether they would necessarily choose to make decisions about their children's development without easy access to professionals – of a type offered during early identification procedures. Equally there is a distinct risk that such a parent-led service would effectively reinforce the 'inverse care law' whereby better educated parents make a disproportionately high demand on the resources of the health system. Health service managers may consider such a distribution to be an economic fact of life and in such circumstances there may indeed be little call for early identification procedures. The dilemma is aptly expressed by Alberman and Goldstein (1970). In discussing a complex model for screening 'at risk' children, they observe that such an approach may be most valuably introduced in areas where there is greatest social disadvantage. In other words, in areas where there are fewer economic pressures there may be no need to actively monitor the population. Again they were not referring directly to speech and language but their position might well be adopted in providing such a service. Essentially there is a need to actively screen or search for cases of children with speech and language impairment in areas where parents do not routinely turn to their doctor or health visitor for help concerning their child's development.

Thus the parent's role is not clear-cut. It is not possible to say that across the board the parent should or should not take the responsibility for early identification. Clearly there should be materials readily available for distribution to parents to help them make their own judgements. Similarly attention should always be paid to their views. Yet health workers should be prepared to undertake surveillance and as a part of this process screening tests can be invaluable.

IS THERE AN OPTIMUM AGE TO IDENTIFY CHILDREN?

There are three possible interpretations of the discussion of the most appropriate age at which to identify children with speech and language impairment.

The first, advocated by Stark and Tallal (1981), maintains that the noise of normal development is so great that any reliable diagnostic assessment before eight years of age is impractical. While there may be some truth in this in so far as it is often not possible to use precise diagnostic categories before this age, it is little use to those involved with the clinical issues surrounding screening. Concern is often expressed before the child is three and so it would not be very helpful to tell parents to wait until the child is eight. Indeed Werner (1969) asked parents of language delayed preschoolers when they had first become concerned about their children's speech and language. The median age given was 2 years 3 months.

The second suggests that any measure should be able to cater for any developmental age. This is essentially prompted by clinical considerations. Children may present in clinics at any time. Having a specific measure which has been shown to identify children correctly at three is of little use if the child who comes to the clinic is 2½ or four.

The third possibility is that primary health workers should attempt to identify the appropriate children at a series of specific ages, ages which have been shown by the literature to be particularly significant in the development of language. These have yet to be clearly defined but a good example would be a vocabulary check at two years by which time children should have made their 'vocabulary burst'. If Werner (1969) is correct in noting parental concerns by 2 years 3 months it makes sense to attempt to identify the appropriate children at this age. Finally a simple test of the child's ability to retell a story at four years has been shown to be predictive of subsequent performance (Bishop and Edmundson, 1987).

In practical terms the real option is between the second two interpretations. There are a variety of considerations which may effect the choice.

1. Developmental expectations. Clearly a child of six months will be unlikely to be referred for speech problems. It is, of course, possible that referrals to speech therapy may be made at this age. But it is highly unlikely that any screening procedure as such would be appropriate. By sixteen to eighteen months it should be becoming clear that language is emerging (see Chapter 1). Any screen at this age – i.e. a measure which is used consistently by a group of staff – would have to be carefully evaluated. The earlier the age of identification the greater the likelihood of over-referral. The optimum age recommended is 2½ to three years by which time it is reasonable to assume that the majority of children will be well on the way to language (see Appendices C and D). Wells (1985), for example claims that by 2½, 90% of children will be able to classify verbally, will be able to use verbs for wanting and making direc. .equests, will be able to express meaning relations such as static and changing locations and possession and will use two constituent declaratives and simple past tenses.

2. Other skills which will be assessed at the same time. It is likely to be an uneconomic use of resources to evaluate each aspect of behaviour on separate occasions. Parents will not be prepared to continually bring their children to a clinic. This then raises the question of which behaviours should be scrutinized at which ages. It may be necessary to choose between identifying speech and language impairment at two to 2½ years and optimally assessing hearing and vision at three years.

3. Previously we saw that parental expectations can vary about

their children's development in general. There is little point in specifying a referral age if parents' expectations do not coincide with the age in question. Herein lies one of the complications of early identification. Advances in developmental psychology and psycholinguistics have led us to understand more about the range of child development. However our understanding is not necessarily mirrored in the expectations that families and indeed cultures have of their children. In many cases this may be a matter of health education but in others there may be cultural explanations for this. It is a largely unresearched area but one which, in the end, will play a large part in determining when parents will bring their children to the clinic.

4. The most appropriate age for treatment. There is now some evidence that speech and language-training techniques can work (see Chapter 8). The problem lies in determining the most appropriate time for treatment. Although there is no reason to discard the 'earlier the better' maxim there is equally little evidence to support it. Clearly any programme for early identification should be dovetailed into such information as it becomes available. Call-up points should allow for appropriate considerations of referral time, waiting lists, etc. where appropriate.

SUMMARY AND CONCLUSIONS

The following points from the preceding discussion should be emphasized.

- There are a set of pre-existing criteria for the development of screening protocols. These include *validity* which incorporates specificity and sensitivity and *reliability* which incorporates inter- and intra-tester dimensions. It is essential to bear these in mind when developing procedures for identifying children with language impairment.
- Parents play an integral role in early identification procedures although there remains considerable uncertainty as to whether it is sufficient to rely solely on their judgement as to whether help should be sought.
- A great many screening procedures are already available. As they become more widely applied and evaluated it becomes easier to assess their relative value.
- Although services often demand that measures should be able to provide an assessment at any age during the pre-school period it is suggested that focal assessment of specific

skills may be a more economic use of resources – vocabulary in the second year of life, comprehension in the third year of life and capacity to relate stories in the fourth year.

- More prognostic data will increase our understanding of the salience of different stages.
- Any screen or procedure for early identification is only intended to help identify those children in need of further assessment. Consequently it need only function in a fairly broad fashion and will not tap the subskills of language in any detail.

To return to the earlier discussion about screening, surveillance and early identification, it is unlikely that a behaviour as complex as language will fit into the rigid framework inherent in the screening process. The truth is that very few human characteristics can be so tightly constrained. For this reason the term 'screening' should be avoided. Nonetheless there is evidence that specific measures may be usefully developed. The criteria for adopting specific measures should be retained as a benchmark and all measures should be held up against them. This is not to say that those that fall short should necessarily be discarded but it does suggest that those measures that are successful should be formally compared.

REFERENCES

Alberman, E. and Goldstein, H. (1970) The 'at risk' register: A statistical evaluation. *British Journal of Preventative and Social Medicine*, **24**, 129–135.

Anthony, A., Bogle, D., Ingram, T. and McIsaac, M. (1971) *The Edinburgh Articulation Test*, Churchill Livingstone, Edinburgh.

Barker, D. J. and Rose, G. (1984) *Epidemiology in Medical Practice*, Churchill Livingstone, Edinburgh.

Bayley, N. (1969) *Baley Scales of Infant Development*, Psychological Corporation, New York.

Bellman, M. H., Rawson, N. S., Wadsworth, J. *et al.* (1985) A developmental test based on the STYCAR sequences used in the National Childhood Encephalopathy Study. *Child: Care Health and Development*, **11**, 309–323.

Bellman, M. and Cash, J. (1985) *Schedule for Growing Skills*, NFER-Nelson, Windsor.

Bishop, D. V. M. and Edmundson, A. (1987) Specific language impairment as a maturational lag; Evidence from longitudinal data on language and motor development. *Developmental Medicine and Child Neurology*, **29**, 442–459.

Bliss, L. S. and Allen, D. V. (1984) Screening Kit of Language Development: A preschool language screening instrument. *Journal of Communication Disorders*, **17**, 133–141.

Borowitz, K. C. and Glascoe, F. P. (1986) Sensitivity of the Denver Developmental Screening Test in speech and language screening. *Pediatrics*, **78**, 1075–1097.

Bryant, G. M., Davies, K. J. and Newcombe, R. G. (1974) The Denver Developmental Screening Test. Achievement of test items in the first year of life by Denver and Cardiff Infants. *Developmental Medicine and Child Neurology*, **16**, 475–484.

Capute, A. J. and Accardo, P. J. (1978) Linguistic and Auditory milestones during the first two years of life: a language inventory for the practitioner. *Clinical Pediatrics*, **17**, 847–853.

Capute, A. J., Palmer, F. B., Shapiro, B. K. *et al.* (1986) Clinical linguistic and auditory milestone scale: prediction of cognition in infancy. *Developmental Medicine and Child Neurology*, **28**, 762–771.

Cochrane, A. and Holland, W. (1971) Validation of screening procedures. *British Medical Journal*, **27**, 3–8.

American Committee on Chronic Illness (1957) *Chronic Illness in the United States Vol. 8: The Prevention of Chronic Illness*, Harvard University, Cambridge, MA.

Coplan, J. (1983) *Early Language Milestone Scale*, Modern Education Corp., Tulsa, OK.

Coplan, J., Gleason, J. R. and Ryan, R. (1982) Validation of an early language milestone scale in a high risk population. *Pediatrics*, **70**, 677–683.

Court, D. (1976) *Fit for the future – Report of the Committee on Child Health Services*, HMSO, London.

Dale, P. S. (1991) The validity of a parent report measure of vocabulary and syntax at 24 months. *Journal of Speech and Hearing Research*, **34**, 565–571.

Dixon, J., Kot, A. and Law, J. (1988) Early language screening in City and Hackney: Work in progress. *Child: Care Health and Development*, **14**, 213–229.

Fenson, L., Dale, P. S., Reznick, J. S. *et al.* (1991) *Technical Manual for the MacArthur Communication Development Inventories*. Preliminary version available from the Psychology Department, San Diego State University, US.

Fluharty, N. B. (1974) The design and standardization of a speech and language screening test for use with preschool children. *Journal of Speech and Hearing Disorders*, **39**, 75–84.

Frankenburg, W. K. and Dodds, J. B. (1967) The Denver Developmental Screening Test. *Journal of Pediatrics*, **71**, 181.

Frankenburg, W. K., Goldstein, A. D. and Camp, B. (1971) The revised Denver Development Screening Test: Its accuracy as a screening instrument. *Journal of Pediatrics*, **79** (6), 984–995.

Gottfried, A. W., Guerin, D., Spencer, J. E. and Meyer, C. (1984) Validity of Minnesota Child Development Inventory in Screening Young Children's Developmental Status. *Journal of Pediatric Psychology*, **9**, 219–229.

Griffiths, R. (1970) *The Abilities of Young Children: A comprehensive system of mental assessment for the first eight years of life*, Child Development Research Centre, London.

Hall, D. (1989) *Health for All Children*, OUP, Oxford.

Hart, H., Bax, M. and Jenkins, S. (1978) The value of a developmental history. *Developmental Medicine and Child Neurology*, **20**, 442–452.

Hedrick, D. L., Prather, E. M. and Tobin, A. R. (1984) *Sequenced Inventory of Communication Development*, Revised Edition, University of Washington Press, Washington DC.

Ireton, H. and Thwing, E. (1976) Appraising the development of a preschool child by means of a standardized report prepared by the mother: The Minnesota Child Development Inventory. *Clinical Pediatrics*, **15**, 875–882.

Ireton, H., Thwing, E. and Currier, S. K. (1977) Minnesota Child Development Inventory: Identification of children with developmental disorders. *Journal of Pediatric Psychology*, **2** (1), 18–22.

Law, J. (1990) Two videos: 'Growing up talking' and 'Trouble talking', available from Health Care Productions, 116 Cleveland Street, London W1P 5DN.

Law, J. (1991) A procedure for identifying children with language impairment at 2½, presented at 2nd International Symposium on Specific Speech and Language Disorders in Children, Harrogate, England. Available from the author at Dept of Clinical Communication Studies, City University, Northampton Square, London EC1V 0HB.

Lee, L. (1971) *Northwestern Syntax Screening Test*, Northwestern University Press, Evanston.

Levett, L. and Muir, J. (1983) Which three-year-olds need speech therapy? Use of the Levett-Muir Language Screening Test. *Health Visitor*, **56**, 454–456.

Masidlover, M. and Knowles, W. (1982) *The Derbyshire Language Scheme*. Available from Ambervalley and Erewash District Education Officer, Grosvenor Road, Derby, UK.

Meisels, S. J. (1989) Can developmental screening tests identify children who are developmentally at risk? *Pediatrics*, **83**, 578–585.

Miller, S. (1988) Parents' beliefs about children's cognitive development. *Child Development*, **59**, 259–285.

Plewis, I. and Bax, M. (1982) The uses and abuses of reliability measures in developmental medicine. *Developmental Medicine and Child Neurology*, **24**, 388–390.

Radway, C. J. and Norfolk, M. (1971) The Surrey Speech Screening Test. *Medical Officer*, 9 April, Vol. 125, 185–187.

Renfrew, C. (1978) *Action Picture Test*, published by C. Renfrew, North Place, Old Headington, Oxford.

Rescorla, L. (1989) The language development survey: A screening tool for delayed language in toddlers. *Journal of Speech and Hearing Disorders*, **54**, 587–599.

Rigby, M. J. and Chesham, I. (1981) A trial speech screening test for school entrants. *British Medical Journal*, **282**, 449–451.

Reynell, J. and Huntley, M. (1985) *The Reynell Developmental Language Scales*, NFER-Nelson, Windsor.

Shahzade, A. M., Becze, D., Christian, S. *et al.* (1984) *Cambridge*

Kindergarten Screening Test, Developmental Learning Materials, Allen, Texas.

Simmons, J. O. (1988) Fluharty Preschool Speech and Language Screening Test: Analysis of construct validity. *Journal of Speech and Hearing Disorders*, **53**, 168–174.

Stark, R. E. and Tallal, P. (1981) Selection of children with specific language deficits. *Journal of Speech and Hearing Disorders*, **46**, 114–122.

Stevenson, J. (1984) The predictive value of speech and language screening. *Developmental Medicine and Child Neurology*, **26**, 528–538.

Stokes, S. (1991) Screening developmental disability in young children, presented at 2nd International Symposium on Specific Speech and Language Disorders in Children, Harrogate, England. Available from the author at Dept of Speech and Hearing Sciences, University of Hong Kong.

Sturner, R. A., Funk, S. G., Thomas, P. D. and Green, J. A. (1982) An adaptation of the Minnesota Child Development Inventory for Preschool Developmental Screening. *Journal of Pediatric Psychology*, **7** (3), 295–306.

Walker, D., Gugenheim, S., Downs, M. and Northern, J. L. (1989) Early Language Milestone Scale and language screening for young children. *Pediatrics*, **83**, 284–288.

Wells, G. (1985) *Language Development in the Preschool Years*, Cambridge University Press, Cambridge.

Werner, P. (1969) Mothers' reactions to delayed language development in their children. *Exceptional Children*, **36**, 277–279.

Whitmore, K. and Bax, M. (1988) Screening or Examining. *Developmental Medicine and Child Neurology*, **30**, 673–676.

7

The health visitor's perspective

Carrie Pollard

In the previous chapter we saw how specific measures have been developed for identifying language impairment. This chapter examines the role of the health visitor, the professional who is the most intimately involved in the process of early identification and consequently the one most likely to be using screening procedures.

The chapter begins with an outline of the role played by the health visitor. The topic of surveillance was introduced in the previous chapter. We return to it again to discuss it here in the context of the current debate in the UK. Approaches to surveillance in other countries will be outlined by way of comparison with the system in the UK. The chapter then goes on to look at the role of the health visitor with relation to the preschool child and finally it turns to a discussion of the specific contribution made to the management of the child with speech and language impairment.

THE DEVELOPMENT OF THE ROLE OF THE HEALTH VISITOR IN THE UK

The first health visitors were paid working-class women who went into the homes to give advice about health and hygiene. By the end of 1905, fifty towns were employing health visitors and in the following year Huddersfield introduced the statutory 'notification of births' which led to the mandatory Act of Parliament in 1915 (Dingwall, 1980). The first training course for health visitors was set up in 1908. By 1918, the Child Welfare Act was passed, requiring local authorities to set up maternity and child welfare committees to take responsibility for the health of expectant and nursing mothers and children under five years of age. The government of the day envisaged a broad training for health visitors in the principles of health and social education. By 1928, local authorities could employ only qualified health visitors. Although there were originally close links with social workers who also began to be employed by local authorities, these weakened when the employment of health visitors was taken over by the National Health Service. When this happened the health visitor's role broadened to include other sections of the population, such as the elderly and patients newly discharged from hospital.

Although health visitors all have a general nursing background the emphasis of their work has always been on the prevention of disease rather than its cure. Indeed the current training in the UK includes not only the psychological, emotional, social and physical development of the individual 'from the cradle to the grave', but also aspects of health which are more often seen as functions of the environment rather than of the individual, i.e. housing, pollution, play space, etc. In this context the principles of health visiting can be summarized as follows.

1. The search for health needs.
2. The stimulation of an awareness of health needs.
3. The influence of policies affecting health.
4. The facilitation of health-enhancing activities.

In the UK health visitors continue to be employed by the NHS and although they may technically be involved with any section of the population, the greater part of their work remains with the under-fives and their families. Health visitors are not specialists in the many different areas of development but act as one of the primary agencies linking the child in the family with outside services, and specialists such as audiologists, paediatricians and speech therapists.

SURVEILLANCE

The picture in the UK

In the 1960s, 'at risk' registers were introduced to identify children who were particularly vulnerable to future disability or handicap. Screening procedures were often targeted at those who were considered to be at risk, physically handicapped or severely deprived. Yet this approach has proved notoriously unreliable. Children on the 'at risk' register were often found to develop normally while a proportion of those who were not on the register were found to be experiencing developmental difficulties. The risks identified were too imprecisely defined and underwent continual revision. By 1976, the Court Report (Committee on Child Health Services, 1976) argued strongly against the 'at risk register' system being used, in part because of this imprecision and in part because it was found to effectively restrict the coverage of the basic surveillance programme. Instead it was recommended that surveillance be expanded to cover all children.

Broadly speaking, surveillance schemes have since been operating throughout the UK. They are for the most part considered successful for the most severe conditions but it has proved more difficult to identify children with less pronounced but nonetheless important problems: mild developmental delays, mild visual or hearing difficulties, etc. Much of the emphasis of developmental surveillance programmes has been placed on refining the various procedures to identify these very children. A distinction is drawn between procedures used for routine surveillance, at which all children are invited to attend clinics at a given age, and **opportunistic screening** at which children's development is assessed as and when they attend the clinic.

A critical review of child health surveillance (CHS) in primary care (Butler, 1989) looked at the national picture and found huge variations in the way in which these screening programmes were applied. Reports from 35 surveillance programmes were examined and it was found that 14 separate screening ages were used between six weeks and five years using 24 different combinations of ages. There are a number of reasons for this variation. In part it is simply a function of the fact that services develop independently. In part it is a result of an uncertainty as to when are the most appropriate ages to identify problems in different aspects of child development. Children with normal development, for example, can localize a sound by seven months of age and this is the optimum point for the distraction test possible (Chapter 5). This type of test would not be appropriate at 15 months by which time most children can discriminate sufficiently to start ignoring sounds made behind them. As we have seen in Chapter 6 there remains considerable uncertainty as to the most appropriate point for picking up the language impaired child.

Butler suggested that a number of areas were in need of simplification. For example, he maintained that screening/surveillance should be rationalized across the country so that parents moving from one health authority to another with their children would know what to expect from the CHS wherever they lived. He recommended that there be as few call-up ages as possible and that this would result in a more economic use of the professional time of those involved.

A shift in emphasis

The surveillance system is extremely costly and during a period of major social restructuring such as has been seen in the 1980s and 1990s these services necessarily come under close scrutiny. Health priorities which were considered to be of concern at the beginning of the 20th century, such as the high infant mortality rate and the need for a fit workforce, are no longer political issues in Europe and the US. This reduction in political interest can be seen in the way that services introduced specifically to improve child health have been eroded. Child benefit has been frozen, cuts have been made in the provision of school meals and the monitoring of the nutritional standards of those meals has been relaxed. These changes are of direct relevance to the work of health visitors who, as we have seen, were introduced specifically to monitor child welfare (Denny, 1989).

One of the criticisms of surveillance has been that such programmes suggest a paternalistic attitude towards the population. Those who hold this view maintain that implicit in the term 'surveillance' is the need for someone to watch over families, as if they are not able to do this for themselves. Currently the emphasis for the responsibility for child care services is shifting from the state to the individual. Thus the World Health Organization defines health promotion as 'the process of enabling people to increase control over, and to improve, their health'. It has stated that 'the starting point in changing lifestyles is to recognise that to a considerable extent health depends on the political, social, cultural, economic and physical environment' (WHO, 1986). This shift then stresses the role of the parent's responsibility for the health and development of the child and correspondingly de-emphasizes the part played by the State.

'Health for all children' and the current debate in the UK

Health for all children (Hall, 1989) was produced as the report of a joint working party review of CHS in the UK. It has made wide-ranging recommendations for future practice in this area. Amongst these the report indicates that CHS should involve health education, surveillance, screening, intervention and prevention. Thus, a programme should not only detect actual, and potential, defects but also provides a framework for the identification of other goals, such as accident prevention. This wideranging approach is termed **health promotion**.

The report recommended that there be a 'core schedule' (Table 7.1).

Table 7.1 Health for All Children – the core schedule

Neonatal	Full examination
Within 10 days	Hips
6 weeks	Physical including hips and weight. Also an inquiry into parental concerns *re* vision and hearing.
8 months	Hearing test, hips, testes, squint test and an inquiry about parental concerns regarding development.
21 months	Inquiry about parental concerns, observe child's gait and that the child is saying a few words.
3 years	Record height, check testes descent, an inquiry into development, hearing, squint, behaviour and development.
5 years	Record height, vision, hearing and physical examination. Also ask for parents' and teachers' concerns.
8, 11 and 14 years	Vision and height. Colour vision at 11 years.

From Hall, 1989.

Although the report has received positive acclaim for the attention that it has drawn to the subject, it has also received criticism on a number of counts. Bax and Whitmore (1989), for example, claim that it focuses on ill health rather than promotes good health. Furthermore they maintain that most of the report looks at physical screening and ignores surveillance for emotional and psychiatric difficulties.

Concern has also been expressed that the core schedule identified above will become the sole provision to the exclusion of other aspects of health promotion. There is a fear that impecunious district health authorities will confine their activities to the core schedule alone, justifying this reduction of services on economic grounds. This is indeed possible. Whereas the usual pattern of surveillance has been for routine physical and developmental examinations three times between six weeks and school entry, and a final examination *at* school entry (Potrykus, 1989a), 'Health for all children' specifically recommends the following reductions.

1. No physical examination after age six weeks, until school entry (except for congenital dislocation of hip twice, undescended testicles twice, congenital heart disease once – but this is omitted from the summary of surveillance above).
2. No measurement of length/height until 3–3½ years, then not again until school entry.
3. No testing of visual acuity until school entry.
4. No testing of hearing except at 7–9 months, and at school entry.
5. No testing of development at all, not even at school entry.

The report also echoes the emphasis on the role played by the parent and in particular the parents' capacity to identify problems in their own children.

In practice, while many parents often do have suspicions about their child's development they welcome the opportunity that routine surveillance offers to discuss their child's development. Perhaps more poignantly it is possible that this emphasis on the parent will effectively reintroduce the inequalities in access to health services identified in *Inequalities in Health* (DHSS, 1980). If parents are asked to make the decisions it is quite possible that disadvantaged groups – those with the greatest need – will make even less use of the services than they do already. Ironically the report which was specifically designed to bring health to all children may serve to limit the access of just those it was intended to help.

The report explicitly does not attempt to determine who should be carrying out surveillance but it does stress that those who do so should not use specific measures. This, the authors conclude, results in the health professional concerned relying on 'box ticking' – administering the test without any real understanding of the process involved. It has been suggested (Barker, 1989) that technical instrumentation should be restricted to those who have a specific training in its use, notably doctors. Health visitors should be encouraged to make use of their considerable intuitive ability and their experience in child development. In addition, training should be offered to provide them with the requisite observational skills and clinical judgement. Unfortunately no recommendations have been made regarding the implementation of such training and no acknowledgement made of the cost that it will entail. Similarly no recognition has been made that the 'box ticking' which is so abhorred is really only a clinical shorthand necessitated by shortage of trained personnel in the first place.

Looking to the future

The future role of the health visitors in any system of surveillance remains unclear. At present, many health visitors are attached to GP practices but maintain their independence through employment by the Health Authority. Under this arrangement they have the opportunity to keep close contact with other NHS employees such as community paediatricians, speech therapists, audiologists, school nurses, midwives, etc. They are also able to work to promote wider public health issues such as the need for clean water supplies, adequate housing, and health promotion in general. The fear shared by many health visitors is that the changing nature of the health service in the UK, in particular as family doctors begin to employ health visitors as 'practice nurses', will mean a parallel shift in emphasis for the role of the health visitor away from public health issues and towards treating individuals on a GP's patient list.

Another possibility may be the targeting of health visiting services to areas in which it is possible to identify a specific need. Although such an approach might be appealing in the sense that it would mean a reduction in the overall cost of the health visiting service, in many ways it resembles the 'at risk' system referred to above which was discarded some fifteen years ago. The worry would be that the role of the health visitors in such circumstances would be restricted only to dealing with the most severe cases. As a result they would come to be seen in a negative light much in the same way as clients see social workers or other agencies with statutory powers.

The shift in emphasis described above has already put increased pressure on health visitors to both cost their work and determine its efficacy. Given the range of services offered it is highly unlikely that the latter can be realistically achieved. For example there has been an increased emphasis on 'data collection' without corresponding attention being paid to what this entails. Thus health visitors are required to specify the number of 'client' contacts without acknowledging the quality or value of the contacts concerned.

A number of statutory changes are currently in process in the provision of child health services. On 31st January, 1989, the UK government published its White Paper 'Working for Patients' representing '. . . the most far reaching reform of the NHS in its 40 year history' (Potrykus, 1989b). As a result, by 1991, the first hospital trusts were established and GP budget holders have begun buying services. In addition, District Health Authorities (DHAs) have started paying directly for services. These major changes are aimed at creating an 'internal market'. DHAs and GP budget holders are now expected to buy services on behalf of the population to whom they are responsible. Hospitals have to set out tenders for any services they provide and to compete for contracts. This means that a whole new layer of administrators is required to cost services, negotiate contracts and to ensure that contracts are upheld.

The Government has repeatedly talked of the prevention of ill health but health visiting and school nursing are not guaranteed as local care services. It is also unclear whether the DHAs have any obligation to provide any surveillance programmes for children at all. The new GP contract, introduced in April 1990, encourages GPs to become more involved with CHS. It is stated that GPs who provide this service will need appropriate training. It may be worth learning from the provision in Germany. There GPs became involved in a developmental screening programme in 1972. The programme was found to be unreliable and the doctors were unrealistic in the time that they allocated for each assessment. Aiming at more reliable results, a standard developmental check list was introduced to the GPs in 1977. They continued to have problems with attendance by low social classes but also found that the GPs refused the supervision required to maintain a consistent service (Drillien and Drummond, 1983).

It is quite possible that similar problems in maintaining standards will arise in the UK. Since April 1990, GPs are able to earn £5 per year for children under five years of age for whom they provide a CHS service. This blanket fee does not allow for the variations in the surveillance programmes offered across the country and consequently what is expected of the GP. Once other costs are allowed for – such as administration, completing claim forms for each child annually, sending out appointments, etc., the fee does little to encourage GPs to make this a priority service.

THE ROLE OF THE HEALTH VISITOR IN SURVEILLANCE – THE INTERNATIONAL PICTURE

There is no exact equivalent to the health visitor in other countries although some do have nurses working in the community in a preventative role. In Sweden, for example, specialist nurses work with both children and the elderly in a preventative capacity, providing a comprehensive service to the whole population. In the US, public health nurses visit some families at home. This service is generally limited to the poorer areas and to specific families where there are particular concerns. There are also nurses working in clinics where children's growth and development are monitored and health advice may be offered. Again, this service is targeted on the poor or those who are not able to afford private health care. As such, these nurses do not have access to the whole population. In Ireland, the public health nurse works in the community as a district nurse, midwife and health visitor. The role is broader than that of the British health visitor although practical nursing tasks reduce the preventative side of the job. For the under-fives home visits are offered, to the whole population at specific ages, as well as weekly child health clinics.

The variation in the role of the professional with the responsibilities of the health visitor at least in part accounts for the variety of different approaches to child health surveillance. Developmental surveillance is approached in a variety of ways in different parts of the world. For some countries, it is probably true that it is simply not relevant. Where there are high levels of malnutrition and infant mortality, and where children's survival into adulthood is a major achievement, developmental levels which are rarely a matter of life and death are of lesser significance. In general, it is only in countries with a sufficiently high standard of living that the services both for carrying out the surveillance and for following up those children who have been referred from it can be realistically made available.

The most comprehensive surveillance programmes are found in Scandinavia. Here, there are well-established systems of child health clinics. Attendance is close to 100% although this must be seen in the context of strong social programmes. In Sweden, up to two years maternity or paternity leave is available and children are seen by the state as having clearly defined rights of their own.

Israel has also devoted considerable energy to the process of early identification of developmental problems, with a total of around 85% of children being screened through their maternity and child health service. The screening includes three to four checks in the child's first year, two in the second year and then annually until the age of five. The checks are carried out by a multidisciplinary team of health professionals. In France screening intervals are at eight days, nine months and two years. Since 1975, in order to encourage a high uptake of these screening tests, attendance became obligatory if parents are to receive their postnatal benefits.

In the USA, preschool screening and interventions have mushroomed since 1961 (Drillien and Drummond, 1983). Current programmes vary from reasonably comprehensive provision in some states to a complete absence in others. The most widely used test for screening language is the Denver Developmental Screening Test (DDST) introduced by Frankenburg and Dodds in 1967 (see Chapter 6 for a discussion of this test). Programmes are carried out both by doctors and by specially trained nurses. Surveillance may be offered by a family doctor but it must be paid for by the client. Some families attend clinics where a nominal fee is paid which covers both their child's immunizations and developmental checks. Availability of such clinics is highly variable although families on 'Medicaid', the free health care system in the US, are entitled to free developmental screening for their children. However, the criteria for entitlement to Medicaid are so stringent that only the very poorest of the population are included. There may also be long waiting lists for referrals to specialists willing to accept patients receiving Medicaid assistance. Families ineligible for Medicaid have to pay for their children's screening and referrals and so parents' income will affect where a child is referred to and the consequent waiting time.

The cost of referrals and treatment will obviously affect the decision of the professionals who implement the screening programmes. They will need to ensure that the family are fully aware of the financial obligations as well as the importance of the children's needs before referring the child on.

Case study 7.1

In Marion County, Indiana, there are some clinics supported by the County Health Department. They offer preventative personal health services and provide health education to all local residents. These clinics are staffed by doctors, dietitians and nurse practitioners. The service is thus aimed at the less well off and each consultation costs $5.

Hank was seen in the Child Health Department at one of these clinics, at the age of two and a half, by a nurse practitioner. He was brought by his mother for a developmental check and for routine childhood immunizations. The immunizations are essential for admission to State schools. Using the

DDST (Frankenburg and Dodds, 1967), the child's speech was found to be delayed. He had never had a hearing test and on discussion with his mother, it was established that the boy's father had also had delayed speech which had required speech therapy.

Before considering the referral of the child for speech therapy or a hearing test, the family's financial state had to be ascertained. Although both parents worked they were still on a low income. Despite having several children, they were not entitled to Medicaid and would therefore be liable for any referral or therapy charges. Taking the family's limited resources into account, the nurse restricted herself to giving advice only, as the family would be unable to afford any further treatment. The nurse suggested that more stimulation would help the speech delay and made some practical suggestions even though she appreciated that the parents' domestic arrangements limited the possibility of the child receiving any extra stimulation. It was arranged that the child's progress would be reviewed, at the clinic, in a further six months' time to discuss possible referral.

Comment: This example demonstrates that there is no set procedure for referring children following surveillance. Access to the referral services is highly dependent on the client's financial situation.

THE HEALTH VISITOR AND THE PRESCHOOL CHILD

The health visitor is the professional with whom all parents of young children will come into contact immediately after the birth and at intervals over the preschool period. This puts her in a central role in relation to the parents' understanding of child development and of their use of the appropriate services.

Health promotion

One of the essential features of 'Health for all Children' (Hall, 1989), referred to above, was that professionals should see themselves promoting good practice in relation to health rather than simply identifying areas where treatment is required. As an essential feature of this, parents and carers involved with the children need to be made aware of normal child development alongside relevant information about diet, accident prevention etc. Of course, parents' need for information and assistance varies considerably. Health visitors must be able to judge the needs of both the 16-year-old school leaver and the 40-year-old career woman who has carefully planned her family. People's experience and perception have a profound influence in their health behaviour (Graham, 1976) and they will interpret evidence of developmental delays in a variety of ways. Their knowledge of the services available will also affect when they first seek advice.

The term 'nuclear family' is often used to describe the typical family in the developed world in which parent and child conventionally live in isolation from the extended family. This may result in a lack of continuity between generations so that each parent has to learn for themselves all about the role of being a parent and about the development of children. This can often result in parents having little knowledge of children and child development. First-time parents are particularly vulnerable in this respect but the problem is by no means confined to them. Even parents who have professional involvement with children may lack experience of normal development. Similarly parents' own relationships with their children can make a realistic assessment of their development difficult. In cases where the child does have serious difficulties the parent has to come to terms with the fact that their child is not perfect before they can ask for help. A health visitor is likely to be a most important link with the outside world in this type of case and is often the one responsible for the referral to developmental assessment centres, speech therapists, etc.

Another dimension to the phenomenon of the modern 'nuclear family' is that increasing numbers of mothers work and have to make use of alternative child care facilities. As a result, the parents' contact with their own children may be quite limited and in what time they do have with their children they simply may not notice developmental difficulties. Such domestic arrangements can also make it very difficult for the health visitor to have access either to the child or to the parent. The cumulative effect may be a reduction in the child's access to professional help should it be needed.

Promoting the use of facilities

Clearly there will be many clients who need additional resources. Part of the health visitor's role is to match up these needs to the resources available locally. A lack of play space is commonly identified as the reason for a child's inability to socialize with his peers. In such cases health visitors may draw the parent's attention to existing local facilities or may help in setting up additional services. This may mean supporting mothers in setting up a play group or toy library and giving encouragement to ensure that it continues.

A close relationship has been identified between maternal depression and the upbringing of the young child. Brown and Harris (1978) found that women with children under five years of age were a high risk group for mental illness. The more stressed the mother is the more likely she is to express anxiety about a child's illness (Bax *et al.*, 1980). Bax emphasizes the role that the health visitor can play in alleviating the isolation experienced by mothers of young children. They are also, of course, in an ideal position to judge the validity of the mother's anxieties.

SPEECH AND LANGUAGE

Delay in the acquisition of communication skills is common. As we have seen in Chapters 2 and 3 this may be a primary communication impairment, or it may be the presenting features of other, more pervasive, disorders (Hall, 1989). Children delayed in this area of development start school at a disadvantage and their identification is a priority. Most parents acknowledge the importance of speech and language if asked and many recognize their children's difficulties when these are drawn to their attention. In some cases this may mean simply encouraging parents to change their behaviour towards the child but in others it may mean a referral on to speech therapy services. It is interesting that parents often accept the need for a referral to speech therapy more readily than they do for other aspects of development.

When considering the possibility of language impairment it is first necessary to investigate the child's hearing. A child's hearing may be quite variable if he is experiencing recurrent bouts of glue ear (otitis media), and a careful case history taken from the parent should identify this. It should be noted that some parents sometimes confuse hearing loss with stubbornness and so may not express any concerns about their child's hearing. Referral to an audiologist may be appropriate if the child fails the hearing test or the parents have expressed a concern.

As already observed, children presenting with poor language skills frequently exhibit very poor interactive skills. In some cases the solution may be as simple as recommending that the child and the parent attend local mother and toddler groups or that the child be sent to playgroup or nursery. Some parents may simply need encouragement to talk to their children because they find talking to a small child difficult or because they do not acknowledge the need to do so. In other cases there may be a need for more active intervention to promote interaction. Again the health visitor is in the best position to judge the level at which intervention should be pitched. As case study 7.2 indicates, this may need to be subject to revision.

Case study 7.2

Cheryl is a 20-month-old single child. She was brought to a local health centre by her mother who was concerned that her child still had a very limited vocabulary. The mother was 20 years old with a supportive partner although she was otherwise fairly isolated as her mother's family lived in the north of England. In all other ways the child was developing normally, being able to dress and feed herself and able to copy her mother's activities in the home.

The mother had no concerns about the child's hearing as she responded well to noises around her. She reported that Cheryl was able to follow simple instructions. At 20 months, it is difficult to perform a hearing test as the child is not yet able to co-operate appropriately. She was referred to an audiologist and a mild conductive hearing loss was indicated.

Observation indicated that the parents understood what the child needed most of the time and provided it without encouraging her to ask for what she wanted. Consequently Cheryl had very little need to use language at all and this, it was assumed, accounted for her limited vocabulary. On discussion with the mother, it was agreed that she should take the child to the local playgroup where there was a great deal of parental involvement. This would enable both the mother and child to socialize with their respective peer groups which would provide an opportunity for the child to use language and the mother to discuss her problems with the other parents present. It was decided, therefore, that the child would be reviewed, at home, in three months time by the health visitor.

After this period the problems persisted and indeed her speech and language made very little progress. The health visitor decided to make a referral to a child assessment centre.

Comment: It is often thought that the unresponsive child is most in need of socialization. This may of course be true, but as Cheryl's case shows there may be other factors involved which need careful scrutiny.

The health visitor is, then, frequently faced with the decision of whether to make referrals of children with poor language development. As already observed, in some health districts in the UK, children are called-up at specific points in their development; in others opportunistic screening is used and children must be observed as and when they attend clinics. In either circumstance the health visitor may simply make a judgement based on training and experience or make use of screening measures of the type referred to in the preceding chapter.

The advantage of making judgements on the basis of experience is that it can be done quite quickly and time is usually of the essence in a busy clinic. The disadvantage of relying solely on informal judgement is that health visitors are given comparatively little training related to child development on their basic course and, of what little there is, only a tiny proportion is devoted to language development. Equally there is often very little opportunity to learn more through in-service training. This effectively means that clinical judgement can only be based on experience and this can take a long time to gain. It is important that such judgement needs to coincide with the expectations of the speech therapist. Obviously health visitors should endeavour to identify children that therapists feel would benefit from intervention.

The alternative approach is to use a specific measure with preset cut off points which allows the health visitor to make an accurate decision regarding referral. In such cases those designing the measure conventionally determine what level of language is considered to be delayed. This approach is ideally suited to district health authorities in which children are called-up for developmental surveillance at specific ages. It is much more difficult to use single measures where children are not 'called-up' as such and where only opportunistic screening is carried out – unless of course the measure in question covers a range of ages. The argument related to 'box ticking' is of particular relevance here. If by 'box ticking' it is meant the use of forms to the exclusion of the application of clinical skills, the point is well taken. Clearly there is no point in training health visitors to carry out such exercises if they could be carried out by someone less well qualified. In reality the complexities of language mean that such an approach would be very difficult to apply. In fact, the health visitor often needs to exploit considerable clinical experience in administering measures of this type. One of the great advantages of specific assessments is that they can provide a focus for the training of those carrying them out. The specialists, to whom these children will be referred, can also be involved in this training. This co-operation helps establish good links between those administering the measures in question and those responsible for introducing and monitoring them. This will be further improved by appropriate feedback from previous referrals. If information is provided about the appropriateness of previous referrals, the treatment given and the follow up offered, screeners become better able to prepare parents for a referral and its implications.

The assessments may also encourage parents to be aware of their children's progress. Their future development can also be discussed, highlighting the most important developmental milestones. In this way, parents can gain confidence about returning to the assessment centre with any concerns they may have about their child's development. It is also an ideal opportunity to discuss how a child needs to develop in all areas. The assessments may also raise parent anxiety about their child's development and, if handled carefully, this can be used creatively.

SUMMARY AND CONCLUSIONS

In summary the following points can be picked out of the above discussion.

- Although health visiting has been of comparatively long standing in the UK it is subject to change. Societal values clearly contribute to determining the role of the health visitor.
- The health visitor is involved in the prevention of disease at both the individual and the community level.
- Many developed countries have professionals equivalent to the health visitor although their role in health care in general and in surveillance in particular may vary considerably.
- Surveillance has similarly undergone change in recent years and remains a hotly discussed topic for those involved in the provision of CHS.
- The issue of the relative responsibilities of parent and state are at the root of the discussion on surveillance.
- Health visitors are an integral part of health promotion, particularly with regard to their provision of services for the 'under-fives'.

- Given how common early language problems are it is no wonder that health visitors have come to play an important role in identifying them. Continuing in-service training is needed for this and other aspects of development in all health districts.

Health visitors need to take an interest in the monitoring of the procedures that they are asked to carry out. They should always know what proportion of their referrals are accurate. This applies to language just as it does to all other aspects of surveillance. It is, after all, health visitors who spend such a large proportion of their professional time applying such procedures. By the same token speech therapists and other professionals working in this field need to ensure that the tasks that they ask health visitors to carry out are carefully developed and that appropriacy of referrals is recorded and fed back to those concerned.

It is no wonder that CHS has attracted so much attention in recent years. Parents and professionals have an interest in providing the most appropriate service for children. As health is increasingly subject to costing it is certain that a price will be fixed on surveillance much as it is in the US and much as it is for other medical services in the UK. It is likely that early identification and screening procedures will be a focus of many future management decisions in the new National Health Service.

Speech and language seem to be a particularly controversial area of surveillance. Clearly a great many children do present with very slow language development. When discussing referral with the parents of these children, health visitors need to know that treatment is available and that waiting lists are of an acceptable length. Similarly they need to be familiar with the nature of the intervention offered to these children so that they can explain the purpose of the referral to the parent. It is to intervention that we turn in the next chapter.

REFERENCES

Bax, M., Hart, H. and Jenkins, S. (1980) The health needs of the pre-school child. Unpublished manuscript available from the Community Paediatric Research Unit, Westminster Children's Hospital, Vincent Square, London SW1.

Bax, M. and Whitmore, K. (1989) Health for All Children: A threat to effective child health surveillance? *Health Visitor*, **62**, 207–209.

Barker, W. (1989) Once again on Child Surveillance. *Health Visitor*, **62**, 174.

Brown, G. and Harris, T. (1978) *Social Origins of Depression: A Study of Psychiatric Disorder in Women*, Tavistock Press, London.

Butler, J. (1989) *Child Health Surveillance in Primary Care*, HMSO, London.

Committee on Child Health Services (1976) *Fit for the Future (The Court Report)*, HMSO, CMND 6684, London.

Denny, E. (1989) The Future of Health Visiting. *Health Visitor*, **62**, 250–251.

DHSS (1980) *Inequalities in Health (Black Report)*, HMSO, London.

Dingwall, R. W. J. (1980) Collectivism, Regionalisation and Feminism: Health Visiting in British Society Policy 1850–1975. *Journal of Social Policy*, **6** (3), 291–315.

Drillien, C. and Drummond, M. (1983) *A Population Study of 5000 Children*, Heinemann, London.

Frankenburg, W. and Dodds, J. (1967) The Denver Developmental Screening Test, *Journal of Pediatrics*, **71**, 181–191.

Graham, H. (1976) Smoking in pregnancy: the attitudes of expectant mothers. *Social Science and Medicine*, **10** (3), 399–405.

Hall, D. M. B. (1989) *Health for All Children*, Oxford University Press, Oxford.

Potrykus, C. (1989a) A threat to effective health surveillance? *Health Visitor*, **62**, 207–209.

Potrykus, C. (1989b) NHS goes to Market. *Health Visitor*, **62**, 70–71.

WHO (1986) *Ottawa Charter for Health Promotion*, World Health Organization, Geneva.

8

Intervention

James Law

The application of an early identification procedure presupposes that there is an effective treatment for those who are identified. This chapter examines what is known about the process of intervention for children with language impairment. It begins by discussing the goal of intervention and goes on to look at a variety of different approaches to treatment. The chapter then turns to the way in which the appropriate behaviours are described and goes on to examine two methodologies which are used to determine change following intervention.

THE GOAL OF INTERVENTION

Before intervention takes place the goal of therapy needs to be identified. A decision has to be taken as to whether its purpose is to provide a cure or to limit the effects of the difficulty. Parents often expect a cure when they bring their children to the department of the speech and language therapist. But for the therapist the issue may be more a question of damage limitation than cure. Both views presuppose an understanding of the process of language development.

The concept of cure derives largely from the medical model and suggests that there is an imbalance which may be rectified by training in a way that an ailment may be remedied by means of a course of pills. It assumes that by directing intervention towards the most salient symptom – notably language – a normal course may be re-established. In addition, it assumes that a language impaired child's use of linguistic structures can be taught in the absence of any strong evidence that this happens in normal development. As was observed in Chapter 1 the communicative development of the child appears programmed to follow a particular course given a basic level of input from the parent.

An alternative approach is to concentrate on improving the child's adaptation to his environment and thereby preventing the development of secondary symptoms. This approach resembles the ecological approach outlined in Chapter 4. It involves focusing less on the symptoms of the child's language development and more on the parents' response to them. It recognizes that the sickness/health dichotomy is inappropriate for developmental conditions such as language impairment. There are sound reasons for adopting this approach of damage limitation. In the first place, focusing on the principal feature of the impairment may be to home in on the primary symptom. While this is an approach common to medicine it is wrong to assume that a spectrum of behaviours as complex as language can be treated in this manner. Working on the very aspect which the child finds most difficult is likely to increase the level of stress and result in a corresponding decrease in the child's capacity to respond. Secondly, the evidence discussed in Chapter 3 gives unequivocal support for a multiplicity of factors associated with language problems. If, in this context, we only focus on the child's linguistic behaviour we may be in grave danger of missing the clinical wood for the trees. Case study 8.1 gives an illustration of this change in emphasis.

Case study 8.1

Laura was three years, nine months when first referred for speech therapy. She had a severe speech problem of a dyspraxic nature. She was dysfluent and tended to use only the single phoneme /d/ as the first consonant in all her words. She was virtually unintelligible out of context and as a result her syntactic ability was much reduced. Her comprehension appeared intact. She was an only child and found mixing with other children inordinately difficult. This was particularly poignant given that she was due to start nursery six months later. She had no history of hearing loss. Her parents were professionals and had very high expectations of Laura. It was clear from the initial interview that they were very disappointed in Laura's progress.

Laura was taken on for a course of therapy which involved repetitive exercises to develop her tongue coordination together with sound awareness work. Characteristically the latter involved trying to pronounce sounds which were phonologically close to those that she was able to use. Therapy also included emphasis on increasing her overall expressive output. Despite, or perhaps because of, the hard work put in by the parents the programme was unsuccessful. Laura became increasingly stressed at the whole process of therapy and would cry when her mother began the exercises.

The programme was stopped and emphasis was transferred to work on symbolic play in conjunction with another child. This required no verbal output and she responded well to it. At the same time attention was paid to including her parents in groups of parents who had children with similar problems. Gradually she built up her confidence with the other children and with it came her expression. She continued to be unintelligible but at least did not avoid talking. Her parents found the shift in emphasis difficult to understand at first. She adapted to nursery well and although her speech continued to pose problems she was able to cope well with the other children.

Comment: The initial emphasis on Laura's speech proved inappropriate. It was more important to work on the child's sociability and the parents' unduly high expectations. This then assisted a smooth passage into nursery. She continued to need help for many years but she presented as a well-adjusted child and her parents responded appropriately to her difficulties. Her difficulties remained confined to her speech and it was possible to direct therapeutic attention towards her speech at a later date.

There is a great need to identify goals prior to the commencement of treatment. These may be changed during the course of any intervention but it is essential that they be made explicit throughout the process. This enables parents, teachers and therapists to share a sense of purpose and this in turn increases the chances of successful outcomes.

TYPES OF INTERVENTION

There are a variety of options open to the clinician when treating a child referred to the speech therapy department for poor language development. The first is of course no treatment at all. Once the decision has been made to proceed, direct or indirect involvement must be selected.

No further treatment needed

For those working in health centres and public health clinics it is important to bear in mind that a referral is not synonymous with a need for therapy. It is likely that a proportion of children will not need further intervention beyond their first appointment. This may be for a variety of reasons. It is possible that the specificity of the measures used to identify the children concerned was insufficiently high. Some children may have improved spontaneously since referral date and no longer need intervention. Others may simply be shy or only be different from other children by virtue of linguistic background (case study 8.2).

Case study 8.2

Eric was two years, three months and from a Chinese family. His parents said that he spoke but said much less at home than did his older sister. He heard both English and Cantonese spoken at home. His parents spoke English and there was no need for an interpreter. They maintained that he was exposed to English more than Cantonese but that he showed no preference for either. When assessed in the clinic by the health visitor Eric failed to respond at all except in so far as he pointed towards familiar objects. His play was limited. He recognized both large dolls and miniatures but showed no real interest in them. There was no indication that Eric had a hearing loss. Similarly his milestones fell within normal limits and no anxiety was expressed about his cognitive development. In this case the health visitor referred Eric to the local community speech therapy clinic. By the time he was seen, eight weeks later, his parents reported that he was 'warming up' a little at home and after three sessions the speech therapist was able to establish a relationship with him sufficiently to suggest that he could use two and occasionally three word utterances in English.

Comment: Eric was clearly experiencing some confusion over the acquisition of language probably as a result of his dual language background. In addition he presented as a child reluctant to participate in the early identification procedure. The fact that his parents expressed concern confirmed the health visitor's suspicion. In the event, the reassurance offered the parents was born out by the fact that Eric coped well in a nursery which he started shortly afterwards.

Great care needs to be taken before reassuring the parent that no further involvement is necessary. Allaying fears inappropriately may be as dangerous as raising undue anxiety.

Indirect intervention

Indirect intervention involves making management decisions relating to the child's communication without directly focusing on the communication itself. One such approach when faced with a language impaired child might be to refer the child for general language stimulation. Care needs to be taken that such provision is not seen as a panacea for all aspects of child's development. Although the results from major experiments in the provision of stimulating environments such as the Headstart programmes in the US have been equivocal in some respects there are clear links between early stimulation programmes and performance at long-term follow up (Bronfenbrenner, 1979). Yet the simple equation of 'if in doubt provide general nursery input' belies the fact that some children are not able to achieve their potential when generally stimulated in this way and many language impaired children fall into this category. The difficulties that they experience in auditory processing mean that indiscriminate stimulation is not necessarily very useful.

Another indirect approach which is receiving increasing attention is the use of parents as facilitators of their child's language rather than offering therapy to the child. In such circumstances the child may not be offered therapy at all and all the emphasis may be shifted to the parent. One such programme is the Hanen Programme from Canada (Girolametto et al., 1986). This provides the families of language delayed children with information to enable them to help their child acquire the dialogue skills that support language development. The principal vehicle for this approach is known as 'the interactive model'.

The interactive model has been developed most thoroughly in the US and Canada (Tannock and Girolametto, 1991). It is one of several methods of parent training which incorporate naturalistic techniques to encourage parents to enhance children's use of language. The emphasis is on communication rather than language per se and on promoting contingent interactions with the child in the context of the child's current focus of attention, interests and developmental abilities. The approach is derived from studies of optimum communication skills which have stressed two factors crucial to language acquisition – active engagement on the part of the child and contingent responsiveness on the part of the child. Three intervention techniques are identified: Those that are **child orientated** such as responding to the child's focus of attention and entering the child's world; those that are **interaction promoting** such as taking one turn at a time and decreasing directiveness and those that are **language modelling** such as commenting on the activities of the child and using repetition and short simple sentences. The interactive approach is currently attracting considerable attention. As yet little is known about the relationship between promoting interaction in this way and promoting linguistic development. Similarly little efficacy work has been carried out to date. Nevertheless it seems to be a positive approach, empowering parents to promote the interactive skills of their own children. For further discussion the reader is referred to Price and Bochner (1991).

Direct intervention

Direct intervention involves focusing treatment on the child. It may be carried out with the individual child or with groups of children depending on the age and needs of the children concerned and the facilities available.

Individual treatment

Children who have been referred to speech therapy clinics are initially seen on their own. This allows the clinician the opportunity to take a case history from the parent and to develop a relationship with the child. Whether or not the clinician would continue to work individually in this way would depend upon a number of factors.

In some cases it is clear that parents need to convey their anxiety regarding their child to someone with whom they have formed a close relationship. In such cases the therapist may decide to extend the period of individual contact to enable the parent to talk through these worries. On other occasions parents may demand individual treatment because they feel that it offers more time for their child. The therapist will then have to weigh up the pressure from the parent with the needs of the child.

In other cases the needs of the child may prevail. In the case of a very shy or reluctant child, for example, individual treatment may prove to be more useful than group intervention. This is usually only a period through which children pass but it is nonetheless important to acknowledge it. Some children are in need of a particularly careful scrutiny and this may sometimes not be available within the group. Thus the elicitation of individual speech or language samples or the detailed video analysis of behaviour may call for extended individual sessions.

Although it is quite possible to illustrate to parents good methods of treatment when involved in groups, this can sometimes be difficult and does not allow the therapist to monitor how far the parent has grasped the process involved. If there is uncertainty in this respect the individual session may again come into its own. As we have seen in Chapter 4 many of the children with impaired language development may also have associated developmental, social and behavioural difficulties. In such cases children may not be suitably placed in a group and the individual approach may offer more to both parent and child. In short the therapist must weigh up the advantages and disadvantages of the individual approach. The strength of peer pressure as a source of motivation within the group may have to be counterbalanced by the individual needs of the child.

Group treatment

This is an approach common to most clinical and education settings. It may be carried out by means of individually devised treatment or it may be indicated by existing treatment programmes. In the UK the 'language unit' provides specific facilities for the language impaired child and offers one of the more direct forms of intervention. Children are usually identified as needing such placement following an assessment of the child's needs. This involves a statement of the child's needs drawn up by all those who have had contact with the child. This includes the parent. Children are offered specific help for predetermined behaviours whether in the field of speech, language or both. At times this involves the child being withdrawn from the class for this purpose, but in many cases children will spend a considerable part of their time integrated with other children who do not have difficulties in acquiring language. The treatment offered in such centres is largely eclectic drawing from specific schemes, e.g. DISTAR (Engelmann and Osborne, 1976), The Derbyshire Language Scheme (Knowles and Masidlover, 1982), The Living Language Scheme (Locke, 1985). Remedial work is carried out by therapists and teachers. The system approximates to a normal school or nursery environment.

Little is known about the relative strengths and weaknesses of different treatment approaches. This is probably not surprising given the demands of both time and resources and given the potential methodological pitfalls which such an evaluation task presents. In one study Cole and Dale (1986) attempted to compare the effects of interactive and direct teaching methods to a group of randomly assigned preschool children with language impairment. The directed group were put on the DISTAR Programme and they followed a predetermined sequence of teaching activities. The interactive approached involved each child being allocated individual language goals and these goals were included in all classroom activities. The result indicated that the language of both groups improved to the same extent.

THREE DIFFERENT METHODS OF PROMOTING LANGUAGE DEVELOPMENT

Three approaches for promoting language use have been reviewed by Schwartz (1987). The first two are adult initiated and the third, child initiated.

The mand-model approach

The adult observes a situation in which the child has shown interest and requires assistance. The adult offers that assistance but conditional on the verbal response of the child. If the child does not respond appropriately a verbal response is given and the child is required to imitate that response. This approach has been shown to increase the verbalization rates of children with impaired language.

Context: At a playground, adult is pushing child on the swing.
Utterance:

A: Say 'push'.
C: Push.
A: Good. [Adult pushes child on swing.]
A: Say push.
C: Push.
A: Good. [Adult pushes child on swing.]
A: What do you want?
C: Push.
A: Great, I'll push you. [Adult pushes child on swing.]

The time delay approach

This involves the adult again observing when the child needs assistance, going to help, but then not actively helping for a period of 5 to 15 seconds, while maintaining eye contact. This technique is useful as a means of accessing previously learned language skills

Context: Snack in a preschool classroom, children and teacher are seated around the table. Teacher prepares snack and displays snack items on table.
Utterance:
A: [Teacher holds cup of juice and looks expectantly at student.]
C: Juice, please.
A: Good, here's some juice. [Teacher hands student cup of juice, and displays biscuit and looks expectantly at student.]
C: Want biscuit.
A: [Teacher notices that student has finished juice, displays jug, and looks expectantly at child.]
C: Juice, please.
A: Say MORE juice.
C: More juice please.
A: Good, here's some more juice. [Teacher pours juice.]

The 'incidental language teaching' approach

Thoroughly discussed in Warren and Kaiser (1986), this approach requires the adult to be ready to respond to the child's initiation. The child indicates that assistance is needed either verbally or non-verbally. The adult then specifically requires a more complex response from the child. The request for a response can take the form of a request, an instruction, a model, a time delay or a combination of these techniques.

Context: In the play area of a classroom. Toys are displayed and some of the preferred materials are just out of reach.
Utterance:
C: [Child points to the blue truck on the shelf just out of reach.] Help.
A: What do you want?
C: Truck.
A: What colour truck?
C: Blue truck.
A: Here's the blue truck. [Teacher hands child the truck.]

These techniques are commonly used in speech and language therapy sessions directed towards the individual or to a group of children. They may equally be passed on to parents.

THE LOCATION OF THERAPY

It is sometimes assumed that the home is the most suitable place for intervention to take place. The young child will be more settled and any interaction will better reflect his or her capabilities. Stevenson, Bax and Stevenson (1982) were able to show that children responded well to a home based language therapy programme in an inner city area. The expressive skills of children who received speech therapy at home improved more than those for whom parents had only received advice. Furthermore the study showed that non-compliant families who failed to show up at clinic did cooperate effectively when seen at home, suggesting that treatment can be successful when programmes are tailored to the needs of the client. Yet it is also true that the home may be full of distractions for both child and parents, making discussion difficult and intervention problematic. Anyone who has tried to carry out a hearing test in a home can vouch for the difficulties in countering background noise.

Where appropriate it may be useful to carry out intervention work in nursery or day care provision. Teachers or care staff will then be able to carry out any necessary remedial work at times when the therapist is not available. A speech and language therapist can provide input to schools by helping to promote appropriate language orientated activities in the classroom routine. In this way the child will receive the necessary assistance without risk of the stigma of exclusion. Yet there are a number of obstacles to school based remedial work. The first is that in the UK speech and language therapists are generally employed by the health services and are consequently based in clinics rather than in the schools themselves. This means that they are coming into the classrooms as outsiders and may find it hard to become a part of the structure of any nursery. This is less true in the United States where therapists are often employed by the public school system. Secondly the size of classes, even at nursery level, often makes it very difficult for the nursery staff to provide specific assistance to individual children. In addition although nursery based work has the obvious advantage of including the teacher it may exclude the parent who would not otherwise be in the nursery. This is particularly important given the need to stress the parent's contribution to the process of change in the child.

The clinic equally has advantages and disadvantages. In its favour it allows for a controlled environment in which there are no distractions for the child and in which the parents may discuss their own needs together with those of their child undisturbed either by the turmoil of the classroom or by the associated responsibilities of the home. Drillien *et al.* (1988) found that the clinic based screening procedure most accurately predicted subsequent performance. Against this it may be difficult for the child to settle in a clinic and the setting may elicit unrepresentative responses on the part of both parent and child. Evidence that the clinic is, in fact, a less appropriate place for working with the preschool child is rather hard to come by although there is some indication that there is an associated difference in performance. Thus Scott and Taylor (1978) found that the language samples of children taken in clinics relied heavily on ongoing and imminent activity while those at home exhibited a wider range of utterances. Olswang and Carpenter (1978) found that it was the elicitor who made the difference and that clinic samples which were elicited by the child's mother exhibited a greater number, though not necessarily a greater range, of utterances. Clearly the clinic has advantages in terms of the use of resources and this is likely to remain a primary outlet for the provision of speech and language therapy.

The decision of where to provide assistance is one that can really only be taken in the context of local resources. In essence there are three options – home, school/nursery and clinic. If we assume that there is equal possibility of access to each setting, the decision to opt for one or another will rest on the needs of the parent and the nature of the difficulty experienced by the child. In reality other mitigating factors often restrict this choice.

THE EVALUATION OF INTERVENTION

There are four stages in the process of the evaluation of intervention (Silverman, 1976).

1. Well-documented observation
2. Careful description
3. Explanation
4. Prediction

Two aspects will be discussed here, i.e. methods of description and methods of prediction.

Methods of description

Historically much of the theory related to speech and language impairment has been generated from single case studies (Broca, 1969; Leopold, 1970; Smith, 1973; Halliday, 1975). Yet useful as these may be from a descriptive point of view it is impossible to generalize their effects without recourse to experimental methodology. Equally it is very hard to reinterpret the data presented in diary studies because it usually serves as a vehicle for the theoretical position of the researcher concerned.

The area which has received most attention in terms of description is that of linguistics. One of the earliest schemes for analysing the child's linguistic output came from Crystal *et al.* (1976) (see also Crystal, 1981). In essence a naturalistic sample of the child's expressive output is taken from semi-structured and free play sessions. The data is then entered onto a developmentally presented chart. The resulting profile can then be used for comparison with that of other children and as a means of ascertaining where intervention should start. The difficulty with this approach is that increasingly therapists and teachers have emphasized the dynamic interactive nature of communication and this level of detail is inaccessible to the linguistic profile.

A second descriptive method which has proved to be of wide application in the type of attachment work outlined in Chapter 1 is ethology (Bowlby, 1969; Blurton Jones, 1972). The researcher uses a set of predetermined and strictly defined operational criteria to describe behaviour in a naturalistic setting. Traditionally recognized behaviours such as rage are broken down into their constituent parts. These approaches have been tentatively applied to the study of communication. Leach (1972), for example, has shown that it is a useful tool for studying the interactions of preschool children with and without behaviour problems. Lytton (1973) has shown that it can be used for parent–child interaction studies. In such cases language is only one aspect of the overall behaviour pattern. The approach has been used with autistic children (Tinbergen and Tinbergen, 1972). Given the emphasis on behaviour it seems likely that such approaches will be particularly useful both for the description of interaction and for the description of 'speech acts' rather than the examination of propositional language. It seems likely that such approaches will become more widely used as the study of the subject shifts towards observing communication skills in naturalistic settings (Lund and Duchan, 1988).

The problem with the ethological approach is that it generally requires observation in completely 'normal' settings. Rating children in their homes the investigator faces a situation which is, as Lytton puts it, 'chaotic, disorderly, unpredictable, uncertain'. In short it is comparatively difficult to achieve reliable results in such settings and for this reason researchers have tended to prefer the more controlled setting of the playroom/laboratory or clinic. And in general this is how the description of children's psychological development has progressed. Some studies such as Wells (1985) have managed to adopt a systematic approach to the study of the child in his own environment. In this case interest was largely confined to the child's expressive output and radio microphones, attached to the children, generated sufficient data. But such examples are rare. Most researchers have opted for the more controlled environment. This leaves the therapist or teacher dealing with the language impaired child with a difficulty in interpreting the extent to which the results can be generalized.

Questionnaires have not been widely exploited in the description of the speech and language impaired population except in so far as they have related to service provision. There have been examples in screening as we have seen in Chapter 6. Superficially, at least, there are obvious reasons for this. There is a fear that the questionnaire provides information only about the individual's response to the question rather than an objective measure of the child's communication. Yet the fact remains that this technique is widely used in both education and child psychiatry. A classic example in the field of psychiatry is the Behaviour Screening Questionnaire (Richman and Graham, 1971). There may well be further advancements in this direction in the future.

Behaviour can also be rated by means of the checklist. In speech therapy such techniques are most commonly used in work with the severely mentally handicapped (Kiernan, 1988). It has been adopted in early identification. Rescorla (1989) has shown that a simple checklist of vocabulary can be reliably filled in by parents. It is uncertain how far such results can be extended to accurately observing other communicative behaviours. There is also the problem of validity. Checklists often combine a variety of different types of behaviour and this makes it difficult to comment on their theoretical validity. This also means that combined scores derived from such checklists need to be treated with caution.

Finally, language is classically measured in terms of standardized testing procedures. Individual children are compared with the large 'normal' population on whom the test was developed. Although specific procedures usually generate less detailed information than a transcription or an observational checklist, they are both reliable and valid. This makes them ideally suited to measuring language in intervention studies even though they are likely to be less sensitive than observations and checklists to significant changes in the child's communication performance.

The descriptive measures selected will be determined by the nature of the task in hand. For a speech and language therapist interested in measuring subtle change in a child's behaviour, detailed observation and linguistic analysis may be most appropriate. If comparison is needed with the normal population a standardized measure will be necessary. Clearly the validity and reliability which are a part of the development of standardized procedures are likely to be particularly valuable for the purposes of research.

The single case study

The methodology for the single case study arose out of the need to test hypotheses generated in descriptive studies. It adds an experimental dimension which enables the researcher, often the therapist, to identify whether the treatment in question is successful once other variables are held constant. Generalization beyond the individual client is established by repeating the process with other subjects. It is argued (McReynolds and Thompson, 1986) that the approach enables the researcher to identify individual's different responses to treatment which in turn enables different types of client to be identified as being appropriately placed in specific treatment regimes. Conventionally, individuals are studied across time and this allows for a close examination of intrasubject reliability.

This approach has two basic components usually assigned the letters A and B, A being the baseline or no treatment phase while B is the treatment phase. By adding further A and B phases it is possible to establish whether improvement in a child's communication skills has been related to the provision of therapy. An extension to this approach is known as the 'multiple baseline' in which two or more different behaviours are included in the same design each with their own A and B phases. Behaviour 1 moves from its A to its B (treatment) phase while the other behaviours remain in the A (no treatment) phase. A predetermined goal is reached in the behaviour 1 which then triggers the B phase of behaviour 2. Other permutations on this model allow the therapist or researcher to use the multiple baseline across settings or across subjects. In the former case, once a behaviour has been established in one client the same procedure is used for a second client. There are a great many permutations within the formula of single case designs and it is this flexibility which has commended the approach to many authors (see Connell and Thompson (1986) for a review of the relevant literature).

Group studies

The use of the group study requires the initial identification of a relatively homogeneous group of children to whom a specified protocol can be administered. This approach enables the researcher to show whether the treatment approach in question has an effect across the group as a whole. If the improvement can be shown to be significant across a group it is reasonable to assume that such an approach can be replicated with an equivalent group with similar results. This in turn allows the researcher to set up hypotheses to compare different successful treatment approaches with one another.

A classic example of a group treatment approach is that described by Cooper, Moodley and Reynell (1978a, 1979). Their Developmental Language Programme (DLP) focused on a range of behaviours related to language development – attention, visual perception, concept formation, symbolic understanding together with aspects of verbal comprehension and expression. These authors compared the performance on the DLP of fifty children seen in a language class with 69 children seen in a language clinic. They found that both the class and the clinic children who had been exposed to the DLP made better progress than children of similar age and handicap having no special help and those having conventional weekly speech therapy. Interesting as these findings are, it is impossible to pinpoint which tasks affect which skills in the children concerned. Given the range of presentations of language impairment indicated in Chapter 2 it may be that there are aspects of the DLP which are more effective for some children than for others.

Other studies have overcome this problem by describing the effects of much more specific intervention strategies. Leonard (1981) identifies a number of such approaches (e.g. imitation based, modelling, expansion, focused stimulation, general stimulation, comprehension based). Of these the imitation based, the modelling and both the focused and the general stimulation approaches proved consistently sound. Clearly the effectiveness of a given approach may depend upon the target behaviour and some language behaviours may respond more effectively to different treatment approaches. There remain too few studies comparing different treatment approaches to the same linguistic phenomenon. Snyder-McClean and McClean (1987) identified 30 papers which documented the effects of intervention on a targetted communication skill. In other words they eliminated descriptive studies. They then subdivided the studies concerned into different clinical groups (articulation disorders; stuttering; language disorders; language disorders associated with more pervasive conditions). In each case there was evidence of the effectiveness of the treatment concerned. Having reviewed the literature the authors conclude:

> But the most basic conclusion we must draw, in view of the weight of the evidence offered by the 30 studies reviewed in this chapter is that early intervention for communication disorders can be effective in modifying the course and impact of those disorders (p. 249).

Furthermore they concluded that direct approaches targetted on very specific linguistic difficulties are more effective and efficient than more general approaches. The problem comes in the extent to which these behaviours can then be said to be generalized. Recent attempts to treat using conversational approaches of the type described above aim to circumvent this problem although without much empirical justification as far as Snyder-McClean and McClean are concerned. Programmes which involved both direct behavioural intervention and back up from parents promote the acquisition and the maintenance of the skill concerned.

An interesting attempt to compute the overall change which can be brought about through intervention is provided by Nye and his colleagues (Nye et al., 1987). They used a meta analysis to examine 43 published evaluation studies using three criteria, notably subject characteristics, treatment characteristics and design characteristics. When treated and untreated subjects were compared across all the studies the difference between the two was 1.04 standard deviations. The analysis of the subject characteristics showed that language/learning disabled children showed greater improvement than either reading disabled or learning disabled children. While most interventions studied were within the school setting the most successful took place within a clinic. Modelling was shown to be the most effective treatment characteristic. Syntactic disability was found to be more responsive to treatment than pragmatic disability, a finding echoed by Howlin (1987). In terms of the design characteristics all the studies were reliably rated as valid.

The interpretation of these results allows for some interesting speculation. It is possible, as the authors point out, that the tendency for the language/learning disabled to improve more than the other groups may be due to the fact that they tend to be younger when first identified and consequently show more potential for improvement. This potential may also account for the fact that younger children generally show greater improvements than older children. It is clear that some studies leave much to be desired in terms of the level of specification given to the client groups and to the treatment offered. Such combined analyses are, then, only as good as the studies that are included in them. Nevertheless the results do suggest both that a level of improvement can be demonstrated and that there is likely to be variation between different client groups at different ages and under different treatment conditions.

The comparative value of group and individual studies

Single case studies are sometimes proposed as a more appropriate way of measuring change. Their advocacy presupposes a number of implicit criticisms of the elicitation of group treatment effects. These have been clearly identified by Siegel and Young (1987):

1. Therapy is primarily administered to individuals, a level of detail which group designs must inevitably fail to capture. Single case studies are, it follows, more directly applicable to the needs of the clinician.
2. Examining the relationships between subjects necessarily loses information about individuals. In the end no single individual may correspond to the mean scores of the group. Groups are likely to sample comparatively small amounts of therapy whereas single case studies are able to reflect much longer periods of involvement.
3. Group studies call for large numbers of relatively homogenous cases. Identifying such a population may delay the

start of treatment and in rarer conditions prove almost impossible to find.

4. Single case studies are inherently more flexible. Therapy can be changed as it progresses much as it might be in the clinical setting.

5. The reliance of group studies on inferential statistics has limitations. They can provide levels of significance for group results, estimations of the likelihood of drawing the same conclusion in replications of the same experiment, but they lose the individual detail which is often so important to the clinician.

While it is true that the overall aim of the group approach is to compare group means it does not necessarily follow that details of individuals cannot equally be extrapolated from the data. There is no reason why the performance of individuals within the group who performed in accordance or at variance with the group mean should not be separately examined. Similarly there is no reason why interpretation should not go beyond the statistical evidence.

The issue of the heterogeneity of groups is one that runs throughout the literature (see Chapter 2). Yet this argument only really stands if it is the intention of group studies to provide information about the individual. This is not the case, at least not in so far as the statistics are concerned. For it is the purpose of such studies to make a general statement about the group concerned rather than individuals within that group. As Siegel and Young (1987) say: 'outcome research will not establish which therapy to use for all clients even if they are all of a certain type' (p. 197). Such group effects will capture something of the tremendous range of variability between subjects, therapists and situational variables. Thus a particular treatment method will on average prove successful with a given client group. Additional consideration will be needed of which child to place in which group.

The whole issue of matching subjects is at the crux of the argument. If it is necessary to match clients precisely and if it is likely to be a virtually impossible task to do, then the rationale for the group must be called into question. If it is possible to say that there are various levels of homogeneity then a more relaxed model might provide a larger sample, from which it would be possible to make more generalizations. A very tightly controlled group sample poses similar problems in terms of generalization to the single case. That is, whether the results are of any use beyond the immediate outcome. McReynolds and Thompson (1986) maintain that this is not a valid criticism of single case designs because the procedures can be easily replicated with other individuals.

SUMMARY AND CONCLUSIONS

- The goal of therapy should be made explicit prior to its start. Those involved need to discriminate between the goals of damage limitation and cure.
- There are a variety of different methods of working with language impaired children. The interactionist approach offers a valuable indirect technique. The involvement of the parents must be balanced so that they see themselves in a position of promoting development, or in the words of Guralnick and Bennett (1987) 'the key solvers of the problems' (p. 368).
- Direct methods of intervention are probably used more widely than indirect methods. As yet there is little evidence of the relative values of the two approaches.
- Evaluating treatment is an intricate business which relies heavily both on observational method and on the selection of subjects. The latter should involve the application of a standardized method of identification of which a screening test might be one example.
- The researcher must consider the value of single case and group studies in the light of the questions that need to be addressed.

At the beginning of this chapter screening/early identification and intervention were noted to be closely associated. It is difficult to justify the former without adequate information about the latter. There is now some evidence for the efficacy of speech and language therapy with language impaired children but there remain a great many unanswered questions. The issue as to whether there is sufficient evidence to warrant the implementation of early identification or screening procedures will be discussed further in Chapter 9.

REFERENCES

Blurton Jones, N. (1972) Characteristics of ethological studies of human behaviour, in *Ethological Studies of Child Behaviour*, (ed. N. Blurton Jones), Cambridge University Press, Cambridge, 3–33.

Bowlby, J. (1969) *Attachment and Loss: Volume 1 Attachment*, The Hogarth Press, London.

Broca, P. (1861) Remarques sur le siège de la faculté du language articulé, suivés d'une observation d'aphenire. *Bulletin Societé d'Anatomie de Paris*, 330–357.

Bronfenbrenner, U. (1979) *The Ecology of Human Development, Experiments by Nature and Design*, Harvard University Press, Cambridge, Mass.

Cole, K. N. and Dale, P. S. (1986) Direct language instruction and interactive language instruction with language delayed preschool children: A comparison study. *Journal of Speech and Hearing Research*, **29**, 206–217.

Connell, P. J. and Thompson, C. K. (1986) Flexibility of single-subject experimental designs. Part III: Using flexibility to design or modify experiments. *Journal of Speech and Hearing Disorders*, **51**, 204–214.

Cooper, J., Moodley, M. and Reynell, R. (1978) *Helping Language Development*, Arnold, London.

Cooper, J., Moodley, M. and Reynell, J. (1979) The developmental language programme: Results from a five year study. *British Journal of Disorders of Communication*, **14**, 57–69.

Crystal. D (1981) *Clinical Linguistics*, Springer-Verlag, Wien.

Crystal, D., Fletcher, P. and Garman, P. (1976) *The Grammatical Analysis of Language Disability*, Edward Arnold, London.

Drillien, C., Pickering, R. and Drummond, M. (1988) Predictive value of screening for different areas of development. *Developmental Medicine and Child Neurology*, **30**, 294–305.

Engelman, S. and Osborn, J. (1976) *DISTAR Language I: An instructional system*, Chicago Science Research Associates, Chicago.

Girolametto, L., Greenberg, J. and Manolson, H. A. (1986) Developing dialogue skills: The Hanen early language parent program. *Seminars in Speech and Language*, **7** (4), 367–382.

Guralnick, M. J. and Bennett, F. C. (1987) *The Effectiveness of Early Intervention for At-Risk and Handicapped Children*, Academic Press, New York.

Halliday, M. (1975) *Learning How to Mean*, Arnold, London.

Howlin, P. (1987) Behavioural approaches to language, in *Language Development and Disorders* (eds W. Yule and M. Rutter), Mackeitt Press, Oxford, 367–390.

Kiernan, C. (1988) Assessment for teaching communication skills, in *Communication Before Speech: Normal Development and Impaired Communication*, (eds J. Coupe and J. Goldbart), Croom Helm, London, 48–63.

Knowles, W. and Masidlover, M. (1982) *The Derbyshire Language Scheme*, Ambervalley and Erewash Education Authority, Derby UK.

Leach, G. M. (1972) A comparison of the social behaviour of some normal and problem children, in *Ethological Studies of Child Behaviour*, (ed. N. Blurton Jones), Cambridge University Press, Cambridge, 249–281.

Leonard, L. (1981) Facilitating linguistic skills in children with specific language impairment. *Applied Psycholinguistics*, **2**, 89–118.

Leopold, L. (1970) *Speech Development of a Bilingual Child: A Linguist's*

Record: Vol 2, Sound Learning in the First Two Years, AMS Press, New York. (Original work published 1947, Evanston II: Northwestern University Press.)

Locke, A. (1985) *The Living Language*, NFER-Nelson, Windsor.

Lund, N. and Duchan, J. (1988) *Assessing Children's Language in a Naturalistic Context* (2nd Edn), Academic Press, New York.

Lytton, H. (1973) Approaches to the study of parent–child interaction: ethological, interview and experimental. *Journal of Child Psychology and Psychiatry*, **14**, 1–17.

McReynolds, L. and Thompson, C. (1986) Flexibility of single-subject experimental designs. Part I: Review of the basis of single-subject designs. *Journal of Speech and Hearing Disorders*, **51**, 194–203.

Nye, C., Foster, S. and Seaman, D. (1987) Effectiveness of language intervention with the language/learning disabled. *Journal of Speech and Hearing Disorders*, **52**, 348–357.

Olswang, L. B. and Carpenter, R. L. (1978) Elicitor effects on the language obtained from young language impaired children. *Journal of Speech and Hearing Disorders*, **43**, 76–88.

Price, P. and Bochner, S. (1991) Mother–child interaction and early language intervention, in *Early Intervention Studies for Young Children with Special Needs* (eds D. Mitchell and R. Brown), Chapman & Hall, London, 225–259.

Rescorla, L. (1989) The language development survey: a screening tool for delayed language in toddlers. *Journal of Speech and Hearing Disorders*, **54**, 587–599.

Rice, M. and Schiefelbusch, R. (1989) *The Teachability of Language*, Paul Brookes, Baltimore.

Richman, N. and Graham, P. (1971) A behavioural screening questionnaire for use with three year old children. Preliminary findings. *Journal of Child Psychology and Psychiatry*, **12**, 5–33.

Schwartz, I. S. (1987) A review of techniques for naturalistic language training. *Child Language Teaching and Therapy*, **3** (2), 267–275.

Scott, C. and Taylor, A. (1978) A comparison of home and clinic gathered language samples. *Journal of Speech and Hearing Disorders*, **43**, 482–496.

Siegel, G. M. and Young, M. A. (1987) Group designs in clinical research. *Journal of Speech and Hearing Disorders*, **52**, 194–199.

Silverman, F. H. (1976) *Research Design in Speech Pathology and Audiology*, Prentice Hall, Englewood Cliffs.

Smith, N. V. (1973) *The Acquisition of Phonology: A Case Study*, Cambridge University Press, London.

Snyder-McClean, L. and McClean, J. E. (1987) Effectiveness of early intervention for children with language and communication disorders, in *The Effectiveness of Early Intervention For At-Risk and Handicapped Children*, (eds M. J. Guralnick and F. C. Bennett), Academic Press, New York, 213–271.

Stevenson, P., Bax, M. and Stevenson, J. (1982) The evaluation of home based speech therapy for language delayed preschool children in an inner city area. *British Journal of Discourse of Communication*, **10**, 141–148.

Tannock, R. and Girolametto, L. (1991) Re-assessing parent focused language intervention programs: outcome limitations and potential, in *Causes and Effects in Communication and Language Intervention Vol 1*, (eds S. F. Warren and J. Reichle), Paul Brookes, Baltimore, in press.

Tinbergen, E. and Tinbergen, N. (1972) Early childhood autism: An ethological approach, in *Advances in ethology, 10: Supplement to Journal of Comparative Ethology*, Paul Parry, Berlin.

Warren, S. F. and Kaiser, A. P. (1986) Incidental language teaching: a critical review. *Journal of Speech and Hearing Disorders*, **51**, 291–299.

Wells, G. (1985) *Language Development in the Preschool Years*, Cambridge: Cambridge University Press, Cambridge.

9

Early identification – a question of science or politics?

James Law

In Chapter 1 reference was made to Gardner's (1983) theory of multiple intelligences. This suggests that there is a variety of intelligences – musical, linguistic, logical–mathematic, spatial and bodily–kinesthetic. But these intelligences are not necessarily equally weighted. Leonard (1987) compares the way in which Western society views language with the way it sees music. Children differ in their musical ability much as they differ in their ability to use language. Yet we do not speak of children being musically delayed and we do not generally refer children who do not meet our musical expectations for remediation. In essence, language is a species-specific domain of intelligence which carries the greatest weight of all the intelligences in our society. Accordingly children who experience difficulties acquiring the skills of language are greatly disadvantaged in the first instance and, as we have seen in Chapter 2, many go on to experience pervasive schooling problems and consequent emotional difficulties.

How children learn language remains a subject for discussion. There are clearly three dimensions which are inextricably linked. There is a genetic component which predisposes the brain to develop a linguistic capacity. There is evidence that aspects of language processing are located in specific areas of the brain. PET scans are showing us that there may be functional differences in the way that language impaired children process language (Robinson, 1991). But language is not confined to neuronal activity. It is closely associated wih other aspects of psychological development and emerges in combination with the other cognitive skills acquired by the child. The child's ability to use symbols is one important example of a complex cognitive capacity which relates to linguistic development. Finally, it is impossible to see language outside the context of social development. As we have seen in Chapter 1 the child is profoundly social from birth and there is a whole year of what amounts to communication training which precedes linguistic development. It is the child's capacity to use linguistic structures in the context of cognitive and social development which is of primary importance both to our understanding of normal development and to our appreciation of language impairment. It is small wonder that we have such difficulty classifying language impairment given the multiplicity of ways that these dimensions may interact.

The issue of intervention will not be clarified until it is possible to isolate different treatment groups, describe their natural history and identify differential responses to therapy. As already noted 'language impairment' is only an umbrella term which covers a variety of different subgroups. We have to go beyond linguistic classification to incorporate specific combinations of cognitive, linguistic and social skills. It may well be that these combinations are not immediately recognizable at the age we expect a child to be speaking. Rather they may emerge at a later stage – perhaps at the age most children start combining words or as they move into the more obviously grammatical phrase of language development. They may then become more clearly differentiated as the child grows older or in some cases the difficulties may resolve altogether.

Can universal screening be justified, given the current status of our scientific understanding? Would it be appropriate to introduce a single screening test across the country? On scientific grounds alone the answer to both questions must be no. If we adhere strictly to the conditions which a screening instrument must fulfil it is unlikely that a single measure will prove sufficiently sensitive. It is possible to use a single measure to generate acceptable numbers of children but this will only identify a group falling below a point on the population curve. It will not help us identify specific diagnostic categories. There is some evidence that all language impaired children start slowly and by three years of age present with an overall delay. At this stage the only reliable subgroups which can be identified are those children with predominantly expressive and receptive impairments. As the child grows older and the nature of the impairment begins to emerge it is no longer possible to speak of a unitary format for any approach to early identification. The problem with a procedure which identifies a single group of children on the basis of a cut-off point is determining that point in a meaningful way. The fact remains that this point must be determined by convention. An argument was presented in Chapter 2 for using −1.5 standard deviations on the grounds that this was broadly in line with prevalence figures. We do not yet know if all children falling below this actually have persistent problems or that children who perform at a higher level than this are necessarily free from language difficulties at a later date.

More work needs to be carried out both to develop accurate functional procedures for early identification and to compare the existing procedures. It is suggested that measures include questions specifically targetted at the areas associated with language impairment as identified in Chapter 3. Thus it is anticipated that linguistic criteria alone will result in extensive over-referral but the inclusion of further discriminating criteria will prove more revealing. Any such procedure should endeavour to establish the level of parental concern prior to assessment.

Nevertheless, despite the comparatively slight evidence directly supporting screening, early identification procedures are widely used throughout the UK (Law, 1991). Few, if any, of these are systematically developed. Yet they continue to find acceptance in apparent contradiction of the evidence. Some would discard such programmes on scientific grounds. Yet perhaps their use reflects values which are not dependent on science for their validity? Those working in the field recognize the existence of language impaired children and recognize the distress that it causes to parents and children alike. Early identification in this context is essentially a practical solution to a clinical problem. The UK remains a comparatively wealthy country committed to public health and preventative care. Whilst this wealth and commitment remain, there is an obligation to address the needs of children with developmental problems. In this context the argument for the continuation of early identification rests on the values of society rather than scientific validation alone. It is possible that these values may be changing in the UK.

However we need to go beyond the belief that early identification is simply 'a good thing'. At the very least we must show that it is not harmful. Some would argue (Marteau, 1989) that the inaccuracies inherent in developmental screening may actually be detrimental to child health for two reasons. On the one hand they may raise levels of parental anxiety unnecessarily while on the other hand they may falsely reassure parents that there is nothing to be concerned about. These concerns alone do not necessarily invalidate early identification. Rather they serve to re-emphasize the need to produce adequate evaluation of screening procedures before such programmes are universally applied.

Illich (1975) suggests that such procedures actually passivise the very people that they are designed to help. Thus they discourage the client, in this case the parent of the language impaired child, from judging whether help is needed. Illich goes on to say:

The truth is that early diagnosis transforms people who feel healthy into anxious patients (p. 49).

Illich's views are partially reflected in the prevailing preference for health promotion rather than screening (Chapter 7). Antecdotal evidence suggests that parents do prefer to make their own decisions about their children's welfare, and that they see the health professional as a means of ratifying those decisions. Parents will often attribute their decision to seek help to an article read in a magazine rather than to any direct advice they may have received. If this is the case, presenting information to encourage parents to make their own decisions regarding child development may be more fruitful than measures applied by a health visitor. In the UK many districts have literature or video material specifically targetting parents (Law, 1990). Such material may be of practical use to many consumers. However it may exacerbate inequalities of access to services. Disadvantaged sections of the community who are already reluctant to make full use of health care are unlikely to be empowered by health promotion alone. It has been suggested that specific screening programmes may be most appropriately applied to disadvantaged areas. While this may have benefits from a scientific point of view it may be unacceptable because of its discriminatory overtones.

It is interesting that while, in the Health Service, the impetus has been away from the application of specific measures, the reverse has been found in education. Thus the recently introduced 'National Curriculum' indicates that there should be a single basic course of study which all children in the UK will follow through their school years. Children's progress is regularly monitored by means of minimum attainment targets at 7, 11, 14 and 16 years. These attainment targets are set by the ministry of education. Much discussion has surrounded the level at which attainment targets should be set and the interpretation of a pass or fail measure. Many of the issues concerning the introduction of the National Curriculum mirror those common to screening and early identification.

It might be argued that rather than identifying children who have failed to reach a certain level of language ability it should be possible to simply promote good practice amongst those working with children. This is suggested by Bradley and Bryant (1985) in their discussion of the early identification of children in nursery who may be at risk for reading and writing difficulties. Yet the difference between learning language and learning to read and write is an important one. As we have already observed, children usually learn language without any specific education. The same is not true of reading and writing. It is not simply a question of allowing adequate stimulation to take place. Enhancing the nursery environment is not the answer for all children. In fact a comparatively small proportion of children attend nursery provision in the UK (24%) and the same is true of the majority of countries (Melhuish and Moss, 1990). Even for those that do attend nurseries the resources needed to offer adequate help to those with language impairment is rarely forthcoming. This then places the onus on external services notably speech and language therapy, psychology and the like. If we accept numbers of children of the order of 6.5% in the preschool population (see Chapter 2) the number of staff available to provide for them is unlikely to be adequate. In summary we are left with a series of questions to which the answers are needed if the process of early identification is to develop.

- Is it possible to determine a pathological level of interaction between parent and child in the first year which can predict language impairment?
- Is the maxim 'the earlier the better' correct in terms of intervention for language impairment? Can we show that it is possible to intervene more effectively with the year-old child than it is with the child of three or five?
- To what extent does language difficulty change across time and does this effect the point at which children should be identified?
- Is it the language level or the profile of abilities which determines severity of language impairment both in cross section and in terms of prognosis? If it is the level what is the optimal cut-off? Is there one range of profiles which does need to be picked up and a second, equivalent, range that does not?
- Which treatments are most effective for each of the profiles identified?
- What level of training is needed for primary health care professionals to use early identification procedures? Can these professionals identify the correct children without recourse to specific measures at all?

- Are simple questionnaires to parents accurate in identifying language impaired children? How do such procedures differ in both their pick up rate and their capacity to predict performance from measures directly accessing the child's language skills? To what extent is this affected by socio-economic status?
- Will the public desire for health surveillance decline as the level of information increases? Will the need for screening disappear if health promotion works effectively?

Procedures for distinguishing one sector of the population from another necessarily raise anxiety as to the appropriacy of the level adopted. It is at this point that society's values and political sensibilities meet with science. The process of referral implies that a need has been identified. In the case of medical conditions such as phenylketonuria the identification of the problem and the need for treatment is not disputed; the presentation and course of the condition can be predicted should treatment not be forthcoming. The issues associated with language and language impairment are much more complex. Considerable progress has been made in the description and remediation of these childrens' problems over the past twenty years but they will continue to tax the skills of the various professional groups committed to their care for many years to come.

REFERENCES

Bradley, L. and Bryant, P. (1985) *Rhyme and Reason in Reading and Spelling*, University of Michigan Press, Ann Arbor.

Gardner, H. (1983) *Frames of Mind: The Theory of Multiple Intelligence*, Basic Books, New York.

Illich, I. (1975) *Medical Nemesis: The Expropriation of Health*, Calder and Boyars, London.

Law, J. (1990) Two videos – 'Growing up Talking' and 'Trouble Talking', available from Healthcare Productions, 116 Cleveland Street, London W1P 5DN.

Law, J. (1991) How are we screening our children? *Speech Therapy in Practice*, **7** (1), 16–17.

Leonard, L. (1987) Is specific language impairment a useful construct? In *Advances in applied psycholinguistics (vol 1)*, (ed. S. Rosenberg), Laurence Erlbaum, Hillsdale NJ, 1–39.

Marteau, T. (1989) The psychological costs of screening. *British Medical Journal*, **299**, 527.

Melhuish, E. C. and Moss, P. (eds) (1990) *Day Care for Young Children: International Perspectives*, Routledge, London.

Robinson, R. (in press) *Brain Imaging and Language in Specific Speech and Language Disorders in Children*, Whurr Publications, London.

Appendices

APPENDIX A   THE EAR AND ITS FUNCTION

The ear is only the first part of the complex mechanism which allows us to make sense of the sounds around us. Its function is to receive the airborne sound waves which arrive at the ear and to convert them into electrical impulses which can then be transmitted, via the auditory nerve, to the brain.

For the purposes of description, the ear is traditionally divided into three areas, each area having a discrete function (Fig. A.1).

The **outer ear** collects sound and channels it to the eardrum, and comprises the auricle, which is the visible part of the ear, and the auditory canal which leads to the eardrum. The auricle has a small function in amplifying high frequency sound and improves sound location. The auditory canal has an important function in amplifying high frequency sound in the range which improves the perception of consonants.

The main function of the **middle ear** is to effect an efficient transfer of energy from the airborne sound waves arriving at the eardrum to the fluid-filled inner ear. Since fluid is much less compressible than air, the power of the vibrations must be greatly increased to be received by the hydraulic system of the inner ear without massive loss of energy. The middle ear acts as a transformer. The eardrum vibrates in response to the sound waves impinging on it and passes the vibrations on through three tiny bones, the ossicles, to the oval window, which is the membrane-

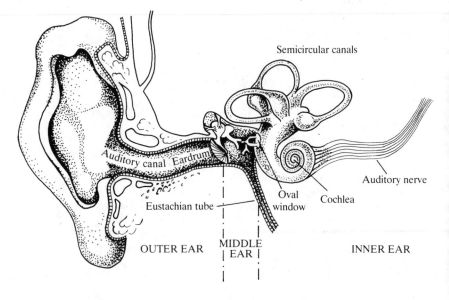

Figure A.1   Structure of the ear.

covered opening to the inner ear. The power of these vibrations is increased mainly by the difference in area ratio between the relatively large drum and the tiny oval window. There is also a small increase in power caused by the lever action of the ossicles.

For the eardrum to vibrate freely and the whole middle ear system to work effectively, the middle ear space must be air-filled and the pressure needs to be equal on either side of the drum. This is effected by the Eustachian tubes which connect the nasopharynx with the middle ear cavities and provide an essential means of ventilation and drainage.

This route for air conducted sound via the ear canal and middle ear is the most efficient means for sound to reach the oval window, with least loss of intensity and fidelity. Sound does also reach the oval window by bone and tissue vibration, but it must be of an intensity of 60 dB to be perceptible. Because of this alternative routing for sound, via bone conduction, the maximum effect of a conductive loss can never be more than 60 dB.

The **inner ear** consists of several fluid-filled interconnecting areas. Since the inner ear has both vestibular and auditory functions and both areas interconnect, some children with hearing impairment also have disorders of balance. The **semicircular canals**, are concerned with balance. They respond to bodily movement and transmit information about body position, via the vestibular nerve, to the brain.

The **cochlea** is the spiral cavity of the inner ear, which receives the mechanical vibrations of the ossicles at the oval window. These vibrations are passed on through the viscous fluid within the cochlea to displace the cochlear duct, the medial longitudinal division of the cochlea which contains the end organ of hearing. The vibrations cause a 'travelling wave' to be generated along the length of the **basilar membrane** which bounds the cochlear duct. This membrane responds differentially along its length to different frequencies and functions as a spectrum analyser. Information about frequency, amplitude and time is carried in the vibration patterns of the basilar membrane. Attached to the basilar membrane are approximately 28 500 hair cells, which are excited by an intricate mechanism responding to the movement of the membrane. Thus information about incoming sound is analysed and translated into patterns of nerve impulses, for transmission via the auditory nerve to the cortex.

APPENDIX B LANGUAGE AND COGNITIVE DEVELOPMENT IN NORMAL CHILDREN

Average age	Language milestones	Cognitive milestones
9–10 mon	Word Comprehension	• Deictic gestures (giving, pointing, showing)
		• Gestural routines (e.g., pattycake)
		• Tool use
		• Causal understanding
		• Shifts in categorization (Habituation paradigm)
12–13 mon	Word Production	• Recognitory gestures in symbolic play
		• Deferred imitation
18–20 mon	'Vocabulary Burst' and Word Combinations	• Shifts in categorization (sorting and touching)
		• Changes in patterns of block building
		• Gestural combination in symbolic play
24–36 mon	'Grammar Burst'	• Active sequencing in symbolic play

Source: Bates *et al* (in press) Early language development and its neural correlates, in *Handbook of Neuropsychology Volume 6: Child Neurology* (eds I. Rapin and S. Seqalowitz), Elsevier, Amsterdam.

APPENDIX C   THE AGE AT WHICH 90% OF CHILDREN ATTAIN A SELECTED RANGE OF LINGUISTIC FUNCTIONS

These are all taken from the Bristol Language Development Study (Wells, 1985). It should be recognized that these figures are tentative. Nevertheless they are the most complete set of data available. The reader is referred to the source for a detailed discussion.

Months	18	21	24	27	30	33	36	39	42	45
Direct request				····	····	····	····	····	····	····
Request permission										····
Exclamation			····	····	····	····	····	····	····	····
Express state						····	····	····	····	····
Verbal accompaniment							····	····	····	····
Content question						····	····	····	····	····
Yes/no question							····	····	····	····
Call			····	····	····	····	····	····	····	····
Elicited repetition							····	····	····	····
Static location				····	····	····	····	····	····	····
Static possession					····	····	····	····	····	····
Classisfication						····	····	····	····	····
Agent action (unspec.)						····	····	····	····	····
Agent function							····	····	····	····
Past simple						····	····	····	····	····
Future simple								····	····	····
Noun			····	····	····	····	····	····	····	····
Adverb				····	····	····	····	····	····	····
Personal pronoun				····	····	····	····	····	····	····
One constituent			····	····	····	····	····	····	····	····
Two constituents (no verb)				····	····	····	····	····	····	····
Subject+verb+object						····	····	····	····	····

Source: Wells, G. (1985) *Language Development in the Preschool Years*, Cambridge University Press, Cambridge.

APPENDIX D   THE AGE AT WHICH MOST CHILDREN DEVELOP SPEECH SOUNDS

There are basically two ways of looking at the sequence in which children acquire the adult forms of speech. The first involves establishing when specific sounds are acquired. Those for English have been classified by Sander (1961).

Average age estimates for the acquisition of English sounds, based on Sander 1961

Sounds	Median age of customary usage	Age of 90% of subjects
p, m, h, n, w	1;6	3;0
b	1;6	4;0
k, g, d	2;0	4;0
t, ŋ	2;0	6;0
f, y	2;6	4;0
r, l	3;0	6;0
s	3;0	8;0
č, š	3;6	7;0
z	4;0	7;0
ǰ	4;0	7;0
v	4;0	8;0
θ	4;6	7;0
ð	5;0	8;0
ž	6;0	8;6

Source: Sander, E. K. (1961) When are speech sounds learned? *Journal of Speech and Hearing Disorders*, **37**, 55–63.

The second involves looking at the way children lose processes which determine types of sounds used. The concept of process analysis is well covered by a number of authors (Ingram, 1976; Grunwell, 1982). There is no data directly comparable to Sander's but Grunwell has produced a table of the sequence with which the processes fade from use in the child's system. This is reproduced over the page. The dotted lines represent the point at which 'almost all children at this age will evidence use of the process' (Grunwell, 1982, p. 228).

Chronology of phonological processes

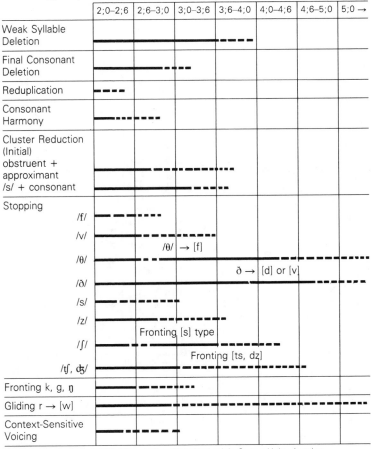

	2;0–2;6	2;6–3;0	3;0–3;6	3;6–4;0	4;0–4;6	4;6–5;0	5;0 →
Weak Syllable Deletion	▬▬▬▬	▬▬▬▬	▬ ▬ ▬				
Final Consonant Deletion	▬▬▬	▬ ▬ ▬					
Reduplication	▬ ▬ ▬						
Consonant Harmony	▬ ▬▬ ▬▬▬						
Cluster Reduction (Initial) obstruent + approximant	▬▬▬	▬ ▬ ▬▬▬ ▬▬	▬▬				
/s/ + consonant	▬▬▬	▬▬	▬ ▬▬				
Stopping /f/	▬ ▬ ▬▬						
/v/	▬▬▬	▬ ▬ ▬▬▬ ▬▬					
/θ/	▬▬	▬ ▬ /θ/ → [f]	▬▬	▬▬	▬▬ ▬▬	▬▬ ▬▬	▬▬
/ð/				ð → [d] or [v]		▬▬ ▬▬	▬▬
/s/	▬▬ ▬ ▬	▬▬ ▬▬					
/z/	▬▬▬	▬▬ ▬ ▬▬▬ ▬▬					
/ʃ/	▬▬	Fronting [s] type ▬ ▬	▬▬▬▬ ▬▬				
/tʃ, dʒ/		Fronting [ts, dʒ] ▬ ▬▬▬	▬▬▬▬ ▬▬▬ ▬▬	▬			
Fronting k, g, ŋ	▬▬▬	▬ ▬ ▬▬ ▬					
Gliding r → [w]	▬▬▬	▬ ▬ ▬▬ ▬	▬▬▬▬ ▬▬	▬▬ ▬▬ ▬	▬▬▬▬ ▬▬		
Context-Sensitive Voicing	▬▬	▬ ▬ ▬ ▬					

Source: Grunwell, P. (1982) *Clinical Phonology* (2nd edn); Croom Helm, London.

REFERENCE

Ingram, D. (1976) *Phonological Disability in Children*, Edward Arnold, London.

Author index

Subject index